Taking Care

A
HANDBOOK
ABOUT
WOMEN'S
HEALTH

Taking Care

A
HANDBOOK
ABOUT
WOMEN'S
HEALTH

Mary J. Breen

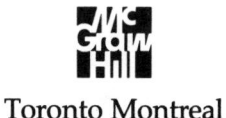

Toronto Montreal

To the best of my knowledge, the information in this book is correct. If you want more information on any of these topics, talk with your public health nurse or your doctor. You could also get more information from a Women's Health Centre or a library.
    This book cannot replace the services of a doctor or other health worker. If you think that you have a medical problem, be sure to get advice from a trained health worker.

This edition published in 1991 by
McGraw-Hill Ryerson Limited
300 Water Street
Whitby, Ontario
L1N 9B6

Cover Illustration by Randy Rozema

1 2 3 4 5 6 7 8 9 10   AP   0 9 8 7 6 5 4 3 2 1

Illustration credits: Bulbul cartoons reprinted by permission.
                      J. Doucette cartoons reprinted by permission.
                      Peanuts reprinted by permission United Feature
                      syndicate.
                      For Better or For Worse copyright 1982 Lynn Johnston.
                      Reprinted with permission of Universal Press
                      Syndicate.

Canadian Cataloguing in Publication Data

    Breen, Mary J.
       Taking care : a handbook about women's health

    Rev. and updated.
    ISBN 0-07-551303-X

    1. Women - Health and hygiene - Handbooks,
    manuals, etc.   I. Title.

    RA778.B74 1991   613'.04244   C91-094334-6

Printed and bound in Canada

TABLE OF CONTENTS

Page

1. Eating Well 1

• The foods you need to be healthy 4
• Special foods for people at special times:
    Pregnant women 16
    Breast-feeding mothers 24
    Newborn babies 25
    Babies from 6 months to 12 months 28
    Children 30
    People with "bad nerves" 31
    People on medication 33
    Women with PMS, Premenstrual Syndrome 34
• Foods to cut down on:
    Fat 35
    Salt 37
    Sugar 39
    Processed foods 42
• How to save money on grocery bills 44
• How to save money cooking 47
• Recipes 50

2. Dealing With Your "Nerves" 59

- Bad nerves and stress 59
- Warning signs of too much stress 61
- Dealing with stress:
  1. Figure out what the cause is 63
     Big changes 64
     Everyday problems 64
     Worrying 66
     Your reactions 67
     Things you can't control 68
  2. Make some changes 70
     Be more assertive 71
     Remove some sources of stress 72
     Change how you react to problems 74
     Change how you talk to yourself 76
     Get organized 82
     Make a new routine 85
  3. Take good care of yourself 86
     Take care of your body 86
     Don't depend on pills 87
     Make time for yourself 90
     Get help and support 92
     Don't expect too much of yourself 94

3. Depression 97

- Common short depressions 98
- Coping when you feel down 99
- Long-lasting serious depressions.. 103
  Depressions caused by health problems 105
  Depressions caused by problems in your
    life 110
  Depressions caused by an imbalance 114
  Using anti-depressants safely 117
- Getting help for your depression 120
- At the therapist's 123

4. Being Active 129

- What being active can do for you 130
- Famous excuses and how to get around
  them 132
- Getting started 134
- Every-day things you can do 139
- Rules for exercising safely 140
- Smoking and exercise 141
- How being active helps during pregnancy 143
- How being active helps during menstruation 145
- How being active helps during menopause 146

5. Controlling Your Weight.............147

- How much fat is too much fat 147
- Good reasons to lose weight 148
- Bad reasons to lose weight 150
- Why some of us are over-weight............151
- Ways to lose weight that are safe............154
- Ways to lose weight that are not safe............156
- Anorexia............166
- Bulimia 167
- How to quit smoking without gaining weight.. 168

6. Over-The-Counter Drugs 171

- Rules for using over-the-counter drugs safely ... 172
- Common over-the-counter drugs:

  Pain pills............176

  Menstrual pain pills............178

  Antacids............180

  Laxatives............182

  Anti-diarrhea medicines 184

  Cough medicines............186

  Cold medicines............188

  Antihistamines 190

7. You and Your Doctor 193

- Your rights as a patient 195
- Your responsibilities as a patient 199
- How to choose a doctor 200
- Why a family doctor is better than the
  Emergency Department 202
- Preparing for a doctor's appointment 204
- At the appointment 207
- Treatment for your health problem
  Medical tests 210
  Using medicine safely 211
  Antibiotics.. 216
  Hospital treatment 218

8. Sex 225

- The sexual parts of your body 225
- Being "normal" 227
- Your right to choose 228
- Homosexuality.. 229
- Sexual problems... 231
- Interest in sex.. 234
- Making love... 238
- Orgasms 239
- Masturbation 240
- Pregnancy 241
- Aging... 242
- Men... 243
- Fantasies... 244

- Sexual assault.. 244
- Sexually Transmitted Diseases (V.D.):.................... 246
  - AIDS and "Safer Sex".. 248
  - Chlamydia.. 255
  - Gonorrhea 257
  - Herpes.. 259
- Pelvic Inflammatory Disease (P.I.D.)...................... 263

9. Birth Control...271

- How pregnancy happens 271
- How birth control works 273
- How to choose the right method for you........... 274
- Common birth control methods:
  - Condoms and Foam.. 276
  - The Birth Control Pill... 283
  - The IUD 294
  - The Diaphragm 302
  - Tubal Ligation.. 307
  - Natural Family Planning 310
  - Withdrawal 313

10. Vaginal Infections 315

- Normal vaginal discharge 316
- Unusual vaginal discharge 318
- Common vaginal infections:
  Yeast infections 320
  Trichomonas infections 324
  Gardnerella infections 327
- Less common vaginal infections 328
- How to prevent vaginal infections 330
- What to do if you get an infection 337
- Getting help from your doctor 338

11. Pap Tests 341

- Why Pap tests are important 341
- How often you should have a Pap test 342
- How a Pap test is done 345
- What the test results mean 348
- What happens if you have abnormal cells in
  your cervix 349

12. Examining Your Breasts 357

- Why you should examine your breasts 357
- When to examine your breasts 358
- How to examine your breasts 359
- Breast lumps 363
- Mammograms 366

13. Menopause **369**

- What menopause is 369
- Common changes during menopause, and
  how to handle them:
  Hot flashes.. 373
  Changes in your vagina 376
  Weakening of your bones: Osteoporosis........... 378
- Less common changes, and how to handle
  them:
  Depression... 382
  Gaining Weight.. 385
  Constipation.. 387
  Stiffness.. 387
  Tiredness.. 388
  Incontinence.. 389
- Taking hormones (estrogen) 392
- Hysterectomy 399
- The D and C.. 401

PREFACE

The YWCA is the world's largest women's organization. Volunteers and staff work together in the YWCA to provide opportunities for growth for women and children. Our goal in the YWCA is to achieve equality, social justice and a safe environment. To do this, we provide programs and services which help women to have more power over their lives.

The Peterborough YWCA has been working to support women since 1891. We now operate two Crossroads shelters for abused women and children. We provide counselling, support and crisis intervention to rural women with the Family Violence Safety Network. We also provide courses and workshops for women and children. Recently we began plans to build 20 townhouses for a women's housing project and a day care centre. In all our work we provide support and information so women can make our own best choices about our lives.

As women, we are responsible for our own and often our children's health. However, when we have health problems, we often have trouble understanding the medical system. We have trouble understanding what doctors tell us, and we have trouble knowing what we should do. One way to begin to understand this system, is to have good health care information. Good information would allow us to make good, safe decisions about our health. Good health care information would help us to choose the best treatment, and to get the best help possible.

However, most written health care information is hard to understand. Even though only one third of Canadian women have more than high school education, most health information is written for people with university education.

For this reason, the Peterborough YWCA is happy to sponsor the second edition of Taking Care. Taking Care contains easy to understand, accurate health information which will help women make good decisions about their health.

We think Taking Care is a useful book for these reasons:

- It is relevant and readable and accurate. A wide range of women were consulted in the writing process. They helped decide the content and they tested the book for readability.

- It contains vital information which women need in order understand common medical practices and procedures.

- It stresses our rights and responsibilities as patients.
- It stresses what we can do ourselves to improve and control our health, such as eat right, be active and cope with stress.

We are familiar with the first edition of Taking Care. We used it in our two Crossroads shelters where our staff and clients liked it and used it over and over. Everyone who read it learned something new, whether she had completed grade nine or university. As far as we know, no other book in Canada contains this kind of easy to understand health information.

We at the Peterborough YWCA are proud to be the sponsors of this unique book.

Lynn Zimmer
Executive Director, Peterborough YWCA
May 1988

Introduction

This book has a long history. It grew out of the work of a lot of people.

The idea for the book began in Kingston, Ontario at a shelter for battered women. The shelter is called Kingston Interval House, and I was working there as a counsellor.

Many of the residents at Interval House had health problems. Several of these problems were the kind that many women have, such as bad nerves and vaginal infections. Other problems were the result of poverty and stress. Others were the direct result of being battered. After talking with the women, we realized that many of them wanted more information about these health problems. It was clear that Interval House needed some handy, easy to understand health books to give to our residents.

When we began to search for the right kind of information, we didn't realize it would be so hard to find. We wanted accurate, readable, and relevant books. We also wanted information which encouraged women to take responsibility for their own health.

However, we were disappointed. We found that most health information is written only for well-educated people. Most of it requires at least grade 12 reading skills. It also requires that the reader know both scientific and technical words and ideas.

We also found that most health information was not very relevant for our residents. It was written for city people with good incomes. It was written for people with much more leisure time than many of the residents of Interval House had at that time in their lives.

So, we decided to write our own. We got a grant from the federal government to produce a book of health information for women. Because I had worked in a women's clinic, and because I had taught reading and English to adults, I got the job of writing the book.

I decided that the book should be written at about a grade nine reading level. This would mean that all the residents could read it -- those who had university education and those who did not. Besides being readable, I also wanted the book to be practical. I wanted to make suggestions which both poor and rich women might find useful.

The production of this book went through several stages. First, I had to decide which health topics to cover in the book. I needed to find out what health information the women were most interested in. To do this, I did a survey. I asked women what health topics they wanted to know more about. From the results of the survey, I chose the most popular topics for the book.

To make the book useful, practical and easy to understand, I met for a year with some of the women I had surveyed. The women in this group read every chapter as I wrote it. They gave me many suggestions as to how to make the book useful and easy to understand. In addition, a doctor, a public health nurse, a shelter worker, a teacher, and several others read every chapter to look for problems. I tried to use all of their advice to make the chapters as correct and interesting and useful as possible.

Many people found the first edition useful, and the copies were all distributed very quickly. Many women said it was the first time they had ever heard much of the information in this book. Because we had more orders than we could fill, I received more money to produce a second edition. This second edition is sponsored by the Peterborough YWCA.

All the chapters have been revised. There is a new chapter on birth control and a new section on sexually transmitted diseases. The revised chapters and the new drawings were field-tested with residents and ex-residents of the Peterborough YWCA Crossroads shelters. The revised chapters were also reviewed by a doctor and several other health workers.

* * * * *

This book is not a complete guide to women's health. Many other health problems are not covered in this book. For example, there is no information here about health problems caused by pollution or by toxic chemicals at your job. Other kinds of medical practices, such as chiropractic care and acupuncture, are not covered in this book. This book is only a beginning.

You don't have to read this book right through unless you want to. One good way to use it is to read the Table of Contents looking for chapters which you are interested in. Or, you could just keep the book handy. Then if you have a health problem, you could look through the Table of Contents. The book may contain some information which would be useful for your problem. Or, you could loan it to a friend, and then you both could discuss it later. Or, you could discuss some of the information in this book with your doctor.

Whichever way you use it, I hope this book will help you. I hope this book helps you to remember that you have a right to know as much as you want about your health. I hope this information will help you understand your doctors better. I hope this information will help you to discuss your health problems with them. I hope it helps you to make good choices so you will be more in control of your health. Most of all, I hope this book will help you take better care of yourself.

Thanks

A great many people helped me with this project.

I want to thank again all the people who helped me so much with the first edition, especially Joanne McAlpine, Mary Pearson M.D., and Ruth Plant. I want to thank Kingston Interval House for supporting the project. I also want to thank the women of my Working Group: Carolyn, Helen, Karen, Sharon, and Teresa. Without your feedback and advice, I simply could not have written this kind of book.

For your help with this edition,

- I want to thank the Peterborough YWCA for sponsoring the project; and, in particular, Barb Morley, Connie McKay, Jean MacFarlane, Kay Roe, Laura Visser, Donna Yuile and Lynn Zimmer. I also want to thank the women from Crossroads I and II who so willingly field-tested both the chapters and the art work.

- I want to thank Joyce Barrett M.D. for so generously sharing her knowledge and experience with me throughout the project.

- I want to thank Jan Catano, Mary Cerré, and Lynn Zimmer for reviewing and editing all the chapters and the art work, and for making such useful and insightful suggestions.

- I want to thank Carol Aird, Gilbert Bélisle, Mandy Bonisteel, Tracy Carpenter, Connie Clement, Janine O'Leary Cobb, Margeree Edwards Ph.D., Anne Rochon Ford, Susan Hubay, Stefa Katamay, Deborah Kennett Ph.D., Robert Kyle M.D., Maureen McKeen, Heather Ramsay, Roma Rees, Lyba Spring and Leanne Tuck who willingly gave me valuable help and advice whenever I needed it.

- I want to thank all the women who have talked with me about their health and their health problems.

- I want to thank my children, Rachael and Gabe, for all their encouragement and support.

- And lastly I want to thank my partner, Craig Paterson, whose support throughout both versions took the form of countless hours of editing, advice, insight, and extra housework. Thank you; I couldn't have done it alone.

Eating Well

1

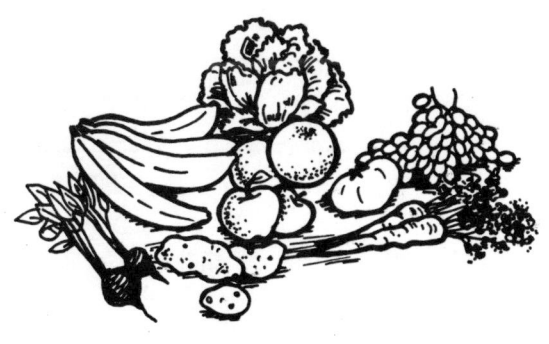

EATING WELL

Eating well is a good way to take care of yourself. What you eat today can make a difference in how you feel tomorrow. What you eat can affect how well you can cope with problems. What you eat can affect how you feel when you are pregnant. It can affect how often your children get sick, and how they do in school.

"How can I feed my kids well with so little money?"

Eating well is important, but it is not easy if you are short of money. However, here are some ways to make the job a bit easier:
1) Find out which foods you need to be healthy.
2) Find out which foods people need at special times. Find out which foods pregnant women, babies and children need.
3) Find out which foods you should eat more of, and which foods you need to cut down on.
4) Find out more ways to save money on grocery bills.
5) Find out more ways to cook so that the goodness of the food stays in the food.

"Which foods do we need to be healthy?"

We have all heard that we need a "balanced diet" to be healthy. A "balanced diet" means that every day we should eat:

- some fruits and vegetables,
- some milk or cheese,
- some breads and cereals,
- some meat or fish or other kind of protein.

Here is how much food we need every day:

Children and adults need
 4 to 5 servings of **fruits or vegetables** a day.

Children up to 11 years need
 2 to 3 servings of **milk products** a day.
Teenagers need
 3 to 4 servings of **milk products** a day.
Adults need
 2 servings of **milk products** a day.
Pregnant and breast-feeding women need
 3 to 4 servings of **milk products** a day.

Children and adults need 3 to 5 servings of
 enriched or **whole grain** **breads and cereals** a day.

Children and adults need 2 servings of **protein** a day.

Think about how many servings of each kind of food you and your family eat. When you do, you will likely notice a couple of things:

- Many of us don't eat enough fruits and vegetables.
- Many of us don't eat enough milk products.
- Many of us don't eat enough whole grain breads and cereals.
- Many of us don't eat "balanced" diets.

You can improve your health by changing what you eat. You can improve your health by:

eating more fruit and vegetables,

eating more milk products, and

eating more breads and cereals.

On the next pages you can read about each food group. You can read why we need to eat more of these foods, and how to do this.

The foods you need to be healthy.

1. Fruits and Vegetables.

Why you need more fruits and vegetables:

Fruits and vegetables are important because they contain lots of Vitamin C, Vitamin A, and fibre.

- Vitamin C helps protect you from infections. Cooking kills some vitamin C. So, eat some raw fruit (or fruit juice) and vegetables every day. People who smoke need more Vitamin C.
- Vitamin A is needed for healthy skin and eyes, and for proper growth.
- Fibre helps prevent constipation. It may also help prevent bowel cancer and heart disease.

Children and adults need 4 to 5 servings of fruit or vegetables a day.

Be sure to eat some fruit or vegetables which are high in Vitamin C such as oranges, grapefruit, orange juice, apple juice, or tomato juice.

Here are some examples of 1 serving of a fruit or vegetable:

- 1/2 cup of fruit juice or vegetable juice (fresh juice or juice made from frozen concentrate.)
- 1 medium-sized apple, orange, banana, or peach
- 1/2 cup of grapes, cherries, or pineapple
- 1 medium-sized potato, carrot, beet, or tomato
- 1/2 cup of peas, corn, turnips, or spinach
- 1/2 cup of coleslaw (Recipes on p. 53 and p. 54.)

Note: Fruit "drinks" and fruit "punches" do not contain fruit juice. Fruit drinks and punches contain sugar, water, and artificial flavour and colouring. They do not belong in this group, or in any food group. Check the labels before you buy, and get real 100% fruit juices.

Note: Potatoes are good for you. Potato chips are not. Chips are very high in salt and fat.

How to eat more fruit and vegetables:

- Serve fruit for dessert with lunches and suppers. Serve fruit on pancakes, instead of syrup.
- Put fruit, not candy, in your children's lunches. Choose small apples and bananas if large ones are too big for your children.
- Give your kids fruit juice instead of pop.
- Serve your children raw vegetables, such as carrots, celery, cauliflower, tomatoes.   Children often like raw vegetables with a dip made from peanut butter or yogurt. (Recipe on   p. 56.)
- Add grated carrots to meat loaf and hamburgers.
- Put lots of vegetables in soups and stews.
- Plant a garden if you can.   Even in a small space you can grow lots of fresh vegetables.   If you don't have your own plot, maybe you could grow a garden with some other people.

The longer you cook vegetables, the more vitamins are lost into the water.   So,
1) Cook vegetables for only a short time.
2) Use a steamer so vegetables are never soaked in water.
3) Save the cooking water and use it again in soups and stews.   Keep the extra in the freezer until you need it.

2. Milk and Milk Products.

Why you need more milk and milk products:

Milk isn't just for babies. Milk products are very important for everyone because they contain **calcium** and **protein**.

- **Calcium** is needed for building strong bones and teeth.
- **Calcium** is needed for keeping your bones and teeth strong.
- **Protein** is needed for building and fixing your body.

Because calcium is necessary for strong bones and teeth, children, teenagers, pregnant women and breast-feeding mothers need lots of it.

All women need calcium because it keeps your bones strong as you get older. If you do not get enough calcium, your bones will become thinner, and they will break easily. This is called osteoporosis.

Children up to 11 years need
  2 to 3 servings of milk products a day.
Teenagers need
  3 to 4 servings a day.
Adults need
  2 servings a day.
Pregnant and breast-feeding mothers need
  3 to 4 servings a day.

Here are some examples of 1 serving of a milk product:

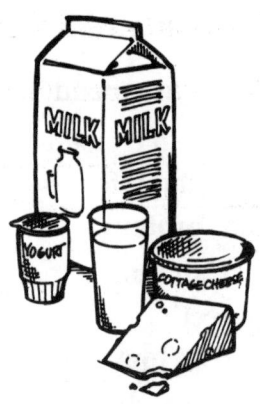

- 1 cup of milk
- 3/4 cup of yogurt
- 1/2 cup of shredded cheddar or processed cheese (Not cottage cheese. It is low in calcium)
- 1 and 1/2 cheese slices

To save money, mix liquid milk with powdered. Mix 4 cups of 2% milk with 4 cups of milk made from powder. Let it stand overnight in the fridge. This milk is cheap and good-tasting. (This is not the right milk for newborns. Please read p. 25.)

How to get more milk products:

- Mix extra milk powder into puddings, sauces, soups, and baking.
- Try some different flavours of low-sugar yogurt.
- Have a glass of milk for a snack.
- Ice cream and homemade milk shakes are good sources of milk. However, they contain more sugar and fat than plain milk. [Shakes from most fast food restaurants do not count as milk shakes. They are made with oil, not with milk.]

If you are allergic to milk, be sure to get enough calcium from other foods. Get a nutritionist's help.

3. Breads and Cereals.

Why you need more breads and cereals:

Many people don't eat enough breads and cereals and pasta because they think they are fattening. This is a mistake. These foods are only fattening when we put too many fattening things on them — such as butter or sour cream. They are very important foods because they contain B vitamins, iron, and fibre.

- B vitamins are needed for a healthy body. If you take birth control pills, you may need extra B vitamins.

- Iron is needed for healthy blood. Because we have periods, women need extra iron. If you have an IUD, you may need more iron because IUDs can cause heavier periods. If you are pregnant, you need extra iron.

- Fibre is needed to prevent constipation.

"Whole wheat or white bread? What's the difference?"

Breads and cereals are made from either whole grains or processed grains. For example, oatmeal is a whole grain. Sweet, coloured, oat flake cereal is a processed grain. Whole wheat flour is a whole grain, and white flour is a processed grain.

Whole grains are much better for you than processed grains. This is because, during the processing, some of the grain is removed. When whole wheat flour is made into white flour, the parts containing most of the vitamins, iron and fibre are removed. Although "enriched" white flour has some of the vitamins and iron replaced, it is not as good as unchanged whole wheat flour.

Whole grain breads and cereals also give a slow, steady flow of energy. Whole grain cereal, such as oatmeal or shredded wheat, gives you energy longer than a sugar-filled processed cereal. This is because your body uses up high-sugar foods very quickly. You may feel some energy right after you eat high-sugar foods, but it doesn't last. A short time after you eat them, you may feel more tired than before you ate.

Try some whole grain breads and cereals. They taste good, and they are good for you and your children.

Children and adults need
  3 to 5 servings of whole grain, or
  3 to 5 servings of enriched breads and cereals a day.

Here are some examples of 1 serving of a bread or cereal:

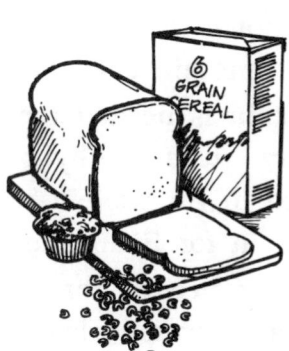

- 1 slice of bread
- 1 bran muffin
- 1/2 cup of cooked cereal, like oatmeal
- 3/4 cup of ready-to-eat cereal, like bran flakes
- 1/2 to 3/4 cup of cooked rice
- 1/2 to 3/4 cup of cooked macaroni, spaghetti, or noodles

How to eat more breads and cereals:

- Buy or make whole grain muffins. (Recipe on p. 57.)
- Serve old-fashioned oatmeal, instead of ready-to-eat cereal.
- Try brown rice or converted rice. Both kinds have more vitamins than instant rice.
- Buy whole wheat bread and rolls. Whole wheat rolls make good hamburger buns, and they are good for sandwiches.
- Add some barley or rice to your soups.
- Try some different kinds of breads, such as rye and mixed grain breads.

4. Meat and Other High-Protein Foods.

Why you need some meat and other high-protein foods:

High-protein foods are very important because they contain protein and iron.

- Protein is needed for building and repairing your body. This is why pregnant women and children need to eat protein regularly. We all need some protein for fixing our bodies.
- Iron is needed for making healthy blood. Because women lose blood every month with their periods, we lose iron. We need to replace this iron. Many women do not get enough iron from their food to replace the iron they lose.

To get protein, most of us think that we need to eat lots of meat. Meat does contain very good protein. However, many of us eat more meat than we need

Eating too much meat can cause these health problems:

- If you eat a lot of meat, you may be eating a lot of fat. Too much fat can cause health problems.
- Meat is expensive. If you spend too much money on meat, then you may not have enough left over for other important foods. A lot of meat and only a few fruits and vegetables is an unbalanced diet.

> Children and adults need 2 servings of protein every day.

Here are some examples of 1 serving of a high protein food:

- 2 eggs
- 1/2 cup of cottage cheese
- 3/4 cup of grated cheese
- a 2" by 1 1/2" by 3/4" block of cheese
- 4 tablespoons of peanut butter

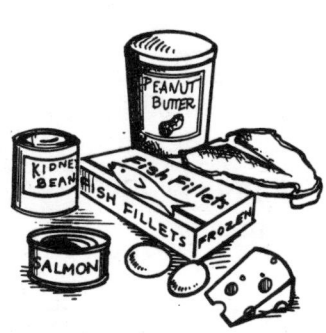

- 1/2 cup nuts or seeds
- 1 cup of cooked beans (Recipe for Chili on p. 50.)
- a 2 1/2" by 2 1/2" by 1 1/2" block of bean curd (tofu)
- one quarter pound of meat, poultry, or fish. (This amount is about the size of the palm of your hand, and 1/2 inch thick. This is about the size of 1 chop, or one large hamburger patty.)

How to cut meat costs and improve your diet:

- Eat less meat. You only need a serving of meat, fish, poultry, or pork which would fit in the palm of your hand.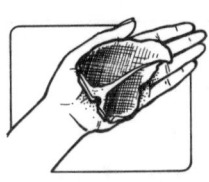

- Buy some non-meat protein foods. You will save money, and you will eat less fat. Kidney beans, peanut butter, bean curd, eggs, and cheese are all good protein foods. And, they are cheaper than most meats.

Compared with other proteins, the protein in meat is the most expensive. You can see how expensive it is by comparing it with some other foods which contain protein. For example:

- The protein in bologna costs five times more than the protein in peanut butter.
- The protein in pork chops costs three times more than the protein in eggs.
- The protein in porterhouse steak costs three times more than the protein in tuna.
- The protein in porterhouse steak costs seven times more than the protein in kidney beans.

If you serve some of the cheaper kinds of protein, you will save money. Then it will be easier to afford the fruit and vegetables and whole grains you also need.

Vegetarians.
Many people eat no meat at all. These people are called vegetarians. You can be just as healthy without eating any meat. However, you have to carefully plan what you eat. If you don't want to eat any meat, check with a nutritionist. Ask your public health nurse or your doctor to refer you.

Water.
In addition to food, we all need water, and lots of it. We need 6 to 8 glasses a day. Most of us don't drink that much. Don't depend on tea or coffee or alcohol for your water. These drinks rob the body of water. You need water, milk, or fruit juice.

Water is especially important when you are sick, and when you are exercising. It helps digestion and it helps prevent constipation.

———————

Eat well, and you won't need to spend money on vitamin pills. Best of all, **you will feel good!**

Special foods for people at special times.

"What about pregnant and breast-feeding women? What about children, and people on medication? Which foods do they need?"

1. Pregnant Women.

When you are pregnant, all of your baby's food comes from your body. Give your baby a good start. Feed your baby well by feeding yourself well.

When mothers do not eat well during pregnancy, their babies can have problems. These babies are often smaller, and they are often born too early. These babies are not as strong as full-term babies, and they get sick more easily.

Some women don't eat well when they are pregnant. This is because they are afraid of gaining weight. **Pregnancy is not a time to try to lose weight.** It's a time to eat good food.

You should gain 25 to 35 pounds when you are pregnant. Women who gain 25 to 35 pounds usually have the healthiest babies.

So, you need to know what to eat when you are pregnant. You do not need to eat twice as much food. You need the same foods as before you were pregnant **plus** extra milk.

Every day you should at least eat these foods :

- **Milk and Milk products**: 3 to 4 servings a day. (This is about 2 more servings a day.) The calcium in milk is very important for building the baby's bones and teeth. If you don't get enough calcium in your food, your body will take it from your bones and teeth for the baby. Besides calcium, milk also contains protein. If you don't like to drink milk, eat yogurt or cheese. Soups and puddings made with milk are also good.

- **Meat or Other High-Protein Foods**: 2 servings a day. The protein in these foods is needed to build your baby's body. The iron in these foods is needed for your baby's blood. Protein and iron are also needed to keep your body healthy.

- **Fruit and Vegetables**: 4 to 5 servings a day. These foods contain important vitamins and fibre. Dark green leafy vegetables also contain iron.

- **Breads and Cereals**: 3 to 5 servings a day. These foods contain B vitamins, iron and fibre. They also provide energy. Iron is needed for your baby's blood. If you get too little iron, you may feel tired much of the time. Many women are constipated during pregnancy. Foods containing fibre can help with this problem.

If you aren't sure how much food is in each serving, please read p. 4 to p. 15 in this chapter.

If you are pregnant and short of money, choose your foods carefully. Choose your snacks carefully too. Snacks like fruit, cheese, nuts and milk are better for you and your baby than chips and soft drinks. If you want to talk with someone about what you should eat, check with your public health nurse or your doctor.

It may be hard for you to afford the food you need. If you are on government assistance, (such as welfare or family benefits), speak with your worker and your doctor. They may be able to get you extra money for a special diet while you are pregnant.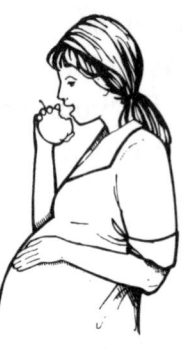

Teenage Mothers.
If you are a pregnant teenager, it is very important for you to eat well. This is because both your body and your baby's body are growing. While you are pregnant, you need to eat well and you need to gain from 25 to 35 pounds.

Many pregnant teenagers worry about gaining weight, so many of them eat much too little. Then they may have smaller babies who are often born too early. These babies have more health problems than larger babies.

Pregnant teenagers often don't eat enough milk products. They also don't eat enough fruit, green vegetables, and iron-rich foods such as red meats, beans and cereals.

Here are some easy ways to eat good food when you are pregnant:
- Have a cheeseburger instead of a hamburger.
- Have milk instead of a soft drink.
- Have orange juice instead of orange pop.
- Have chili instead of a hot dog.
- Have ice cream instead of cake.
- Have whole wheat crackers and cheese instead of chips.
- Have a peanut butter and honey sandwich instead of a donut.

Eat well and have a healthy baby.

Things to Avoid During Pregnancy.

Almost everything you eat or drink can be passed on to your baby. No drug is absolutely safe for an unborn baby, and some can harm it. Don't take any chances. Don't take any drugs.

Here are some drugs to avoid when you are pregnant:

Alcohol.

Alcohol is a drug. It passes from your bloodstream into your baby's. In large amounts, alcohol can seriously harm your unborn baby. No one knows how much alcohol is safe for a pregnant woman to drink. So, the less you drink the better. When you are pregnant, it's best not to drink any alcohol at all.

Cigarettes.

Cigarettes contain nicotine, which is a drug. Cigarettes are harmful both to adults and babies. You may know that smoking can hurt <u>you</u>, but you may not know that smoking can also hurt your baby.

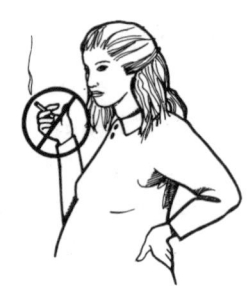

This is how smoking hurts your baby:

Babies need a good supply of oxygen and food to be healthy. They get this oxygen and food through their mother's blood. When pregnant women smoke, chemicals in the smoke affect their blood.

1. These chemicals make both the mother's blood and the baby's blood less able to carry oxygen.

2. The chemicals make the mother's blood flow more slowly. This means that less food and oxygen can reach the baby.

Because the babies of women who smoke get less food and oxygen, these babies are often smaller. They are more often born too soon, and they have a higher risk of dying early in life. Women who smoke also have more miscarriages. After birth, babies who live with smokers have twice as much bronchitis and pneumonia as babies who live with nonsmokers.

If you are pregnant, the sooner you quit smoking the better off your baby will be. Try to quit for the sake of your baby. If you can't quit, at least cut down while you are pregnant. Quitting smoking is one of the best gifts you can give to your baby.

Drugs and Medicines.

Check with your doctor before you take any drugs or medicines:

- Check with your doctor before you take drugs you can buy without a prescription, for example: cough medicine, aspirin, and laxatives.
- Check with your doctor before you take prescription drugs. (If your doctor gives you a prescription, make sure that she or he knows you are pregnant. Make sure the drug is safe for pregnant women. Never take someone else's prescription.)
- Don't take tranquillizers or sleeping pills.
- Don't take diet pills.
- Don't take street drugs, such as marijuana or cocaine or heroin.

Caffeine.

Caffeine is another common drug. Caffeine is found in coffee and tea. It is also in chocolate, in cola drinks, and in some medicines such as headache pills. Caffeine is a stimulant, and it affects your baby as well as you. It's a good idea to cut down on caffeine while you are pregnant.

Don't take any chances with drugs when you are pregnant.

Morning-sickness.

Many women are morning-sick during the first few months. If you have morning sickness, here are some ways to control it:

- Eat dry crackers or cereal 15 minutes before you get out of bed. Put the food by your bed at night. In the morning, eat it slowly before you get out of bed.
- Avoid large meals. Instead, eat lots of small meals.
- Avoid coffee.
- Avoid fried or fatty foods.
- Eat bland foods, such as puddings and yogurt and bananas.
- Apple, orange or tomato juice may help you get rid of your morning sickness. However, for some women, juice makes it worse.

2. Breast-Feeding Mothers.

If you eat well, you will be able to produce lots of good breast milk for your baby. If you eat well, you will stay healthy too.

While you are breast-feeding, you need plenty of liquids. You also need the same foods as when you were pregnant:

- Milk and Milk products: 3 to 4 servings a day.
- Meat or Other High-Protein Foods: 2 servings a day.
- Fruit and Vegetables: 4 to 5 servings a day.
- Breads and Cereals: 3 to 5 servings a day.

If you want to know more about why these foods are important, please read p. 4 to p. 15 in this chapter.

Drugs. Both caffeine and nicotine are passed on to your baby through your breast milk. Coffee, tea, some cola drinks and some drugs contain caffeine. Caffeine in breast milk makes some babies jittery. Nicotine makes your baby's heart beat faster. It also makes your baby's blood less able to carry oxygen. It is very important to cut down on smoking while you are breast-feeding.

Breast-feeding mothers must not take certain drugs. If your doctor gives you a drug while you are breast-feeding, make sure it is safe.

3. Newborn Babies.

Babies must have good food, especially in their first two years. If they don't get good basic food, it can permanently affect their health, and how well they can learn. This isn't meant to scare you, but to tell you how important it is to feed your baby well.

During their first six months, babies only need milk. The best milk for babies is breast milk.

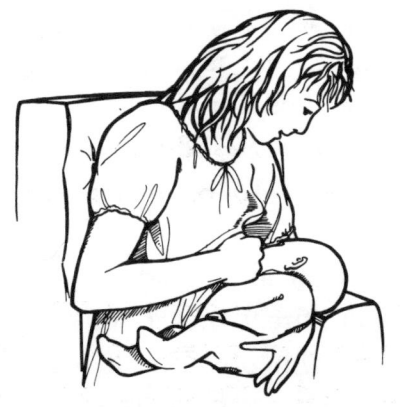

Breast-Feeding.
Nearly all women can breast-feed and many do. There are several good reasons to breast feed.

Breast-feeding is good for your baby because:
- Breast milk contains the right mixture of foods for a human baby.
- Babies can digest breast milk more easily than any other kind.
- Breast-fed babies get fewer infections, such as colds.
- Breast-fed babies also have fewer allergies.

Breast-feeding is good for you because:
- Breast milk is cheap. There are no bottles or formula to buy. In 1991, the cost of ready-to-feed formula for half a year is about $890.00. However, the cost of extra food for the breast-feeding mother is only about $266.00. Ready-to-feed formula costs over three times more than breast milk.
- Breast milk is clean and handy. It is always at the right temperature. Breast milk is also always ready-to-serve. With breast milk you don't have to worry about mixing formula correctly in the middle of the night.
- Breast milk takes no time to prepare. If you breast-feed, you will save hours of formula-mixing time.
- Breast-feeding helps you and your baby to be extra close.

Think carefully about whether you are going to breast-feed or not. You could give it a try for a while. Even if you don't want to breast-feed for a long time, try breast-feeding for one month. Even one month of breast-feeding will help to protect your baby from getting sick during its early months.

If you want help with breast-feeding, you could contact the La Leche League in your area. This group gives free information and support to any breast-feeding mother. You can get help over the telephone, or you can go to one of their meetings. They could help you with problems such as sore nipples, or how to keep on breast-feeding after you go back to work. You can get the number for La Leche League from a public health unit, from a hospital, or from the phone book.

Formula Feeding.
If you decide not to breast-feed, the next best thing is store-bought formula. Formula is much better than regular milk for small babies.

- Babies should <u>not</u> have regular milk until they are at least 6 months old.
- After 6 months, they need <u>homo</u> milk until they are at least 12 months old.
- Do not give them skim or 2% milk before they are at least 12 months old. Babies need the fat in homo milk.

4. Babies from 6 Months to 12 Months.

For their first six months, babies only need milk. When they are between 4 and 6 months old, they can start on some solid foods. Talk to your public health nurse or your doctor about giving your baby solid food. They can give you advice about which foods to give your baby at each age.

You don't need to buy all your baby's food. You can make some of it. If you make your own, you will save money.

Making Your Own Baby Food.

1. Choose fresh or frozen fruit or vegetables.
2. Choose fresh meat or fish, not canned. Canned meats contain too much salt.
3. Do not add any sugar, salt or fat to the food. (Extra salt and sugar are not good for babies.)
4. Use very clean pots and utensils. Make sure your hands are clean. Wash the fruit or vegetables well.
5. Cook the food. When you are cooking fruit or vegetables, use a small amount of water. Don't cook it for very long.

6. Then blend it in a blender or a baby food grinder.

7. Then put the food in the fridge right away. Don't keep it any longer than 3 days in the fridge.

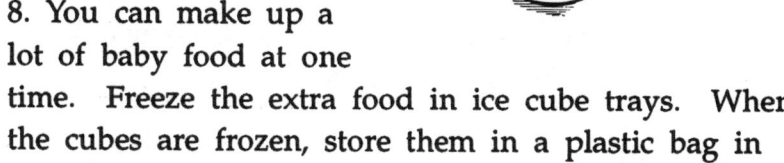

8. You can make up a lot of baby food at one time. Freeze the extra food in ice cube trays. When the cubes are frozen, store them in a plastic bag in the freezer.

9. When you need some, thaw the cubes one at a time. One cube of food, thawed, will serve a small baby.

If you aren't sure how to do this, check with your public health nurse.

Babies don't need sweet desserts. Babies don't need sugar. Instead, give your baby some plain yogurt, or mashed up soft banana.

If your baby is thirsty, give her water, milk or juice mixed with a little water. Don't give babies pop or drinks made from powdered crystals. Too many sweetened drinks, especially at bed-time, can cause tooth decay.

5. Children.

Children need good food to help them grow. They also need good food to give them energy to be active, and to help them fight infections. Healthy children don't get sick as often. When they do get sick, they don't get as sick. They also get better more quickly.

When you choose snacks for your kids, remember that most kids like healthy snacks such as:

- fresh fruit
- raw vegetables
- milk
- crackers
- muffins
- fruit juice
- cheese
- popcorn

Remember: Children can easily choke on hard foods. Always stay with children when they are eating popcorn, nuts, and hard, raw vegetables. Nuts are very dangerous. Don't give them to children under four years old. When you give them to older children, tell them that they must chew them very well.

Fruit is not as expensive as you may think. If you compare the price of fruit with the price of treats, you will see how cheap some fruit really is.

This list shows the 1991 Ontario prices of the same weight of different foods. (1 kilogram = just over 2 pounds.)

1 kilogram of bananas costs about $1.50
1 kilogram of apples costs about $2.00
1 kilogram of oatmeal cookies costs about $7.50
1 kilogram of potato chips costs about $13.00
1 kilogram of chocolate bars costs about $16.50

Sweets are OK now and again. But, be sure to cover the basics first. Cover the basics before you spend your hard-earned money on food that no one really needs.

6. People with "Bad Nerves".

If you have "bad nerves", you can make them worse by what you eat.

Here are some ways to help your nerves by changing what you eat:
• Cut down on caffeine. Caffeine is a stimulant. If you get too much of it, you may become jittery, cranky and have trouble sleeping. There is caffeine in coffee, tea, chocolate and cola drinks.

If you feel jumpy or cranky, try cutting down on caffeine. See if it makes a difference in how you feel. Don't drink more than 4 cups a day. Instead, try decaffeinated coffee, weaker tea and other non-caffeine drinks, especially in the evening.

If your kids are jumpy, they may be getting too much caffeine too. For a small child, one 12-ounce bottle of cola has the same effect as 4 cups of coffee for an adult! Give them white milk or unsweetened fruit juice instead.

- Drink plenty of non-caffeine drinks, such as water, juice and milk. Avoid drinking much alcohol.

- If you have trouble sleeping, get some exercise. Cut down on caffeine drinks in the evening. Don't take sleeping pills. Instead, have a warm cup of milk before bed.
When you are tired and tense, go for a walk. A ten-minute walk can make you feel better. You will be less tense, and you will have more energy than if you ate a candy bar.

- Remember to eat well, and eat regularly. Three small meals are much better than one large one.

7. People on Medication.

Some people have to take medication on a regular basis.

If you are taking medication, ask your doctor or your druggist for advice about what you should eat.
- You may have to avoid certain foods. Some medicines do not work well if you eat certain foods. If you feel sick or uncomfortable after you eat certain foods, be sure to tell your doctor.
- You may have to eat more of certain foods. Some medicines work better if you eat certain foods.
- You should eat a good diet when you are on any medication. A good diet will help to prevent the medicine from using up your body's supply of vitamins and minerals.

Birth Control Pills.
If you take the Pill, it is important for you to eat well. If you are on the Pill, you need to eat more of these foods which contain vitamin B:
- more protein foods (hamburger, peanuts, eggs)
- more oranges and grapefruit (Take your Pill with orange juice.)
- more whole grain breads and cereals
- more dark green vegetables (broccoli, parsley)

8. Women with PMS (Premenstrual Syndrome).

PMS stands for all the changes which many women notice every month before their periods. Many women have PMS, but it is not the same for all women. Some women have headaches and become bloated. Others feel cranky, or tearful, or depressed. Others crave special foods.

If you have PMS, it may improve if you change what you eat.

- Eat more whole grain breads and cereals, and more fruits and vegetables.
- Eat much less sugar, and much less salt.
- Drink much less alcohol, and much less caffeine.
- Drink much more water.
- Eat regularly. Don't go without food for a long time.
- Exercise more.

Many women have sore breasts in the week before their period. Your breasts will be less sore and swollen if you:

- eat less salt
- eat less food containing fat
- avoid caffeine. There is caffeine in coffee, tea, colas, chocolate, and in some cold remedies and pain pills.

"What foods should I cut down on?"

You may not be rich, but you may be eating rich, expensive and unhealthy foods.

You can improve your family's health by eating:

less fat

less salt

less sugar

less processed food.

Foods to cut down on.

Eating less fat.

"Why should I eat less fat?"

Most of us eat far too much fat. Eating too much fat can cause many health problems.

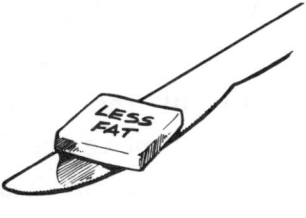

- Too much fat increases your chances of getting breast cancer and bowel cancer.
- Too much fat also increases your chances of having high blood pressure.
- Too much fat increases your chances of getting fat. Fat is high in calories. Unless you are very active, if you eat a lot of fat, you will get fat. And, people who are fat are more likely to get high blood pressure and diabetes.

"How do I eat less fat?"

- Eat less sour cream, cream cheese, butter, margarine, mayonnaise and salad dressings.
- Avoid cheesecake, wieners, cold cuts, deep-fried foods, potato chips, gravy, donuts, and pastries. All of these foods contain lots of hidden fat.
- Eat less "fast food", such as fish and chips, hot dogs, and shakes. For example, a piece of deep-fried chicken contains 5 times more fat than a piece broiled with the skin removed. Fast food shakes are made with oil, not milk.
- Serve more chicken and fish than red meat. Always remove the skin from chicken, before you cook it. The skin contains a lot of fat.
- Trim off the fat of meat before you cook it. You can't remove the fat in hamburger, but you can cook it at low heat, and drain the fat off as it melts. If it sticks, add a little water, not more fat.
- Don't use fat for cooking. Buy a non-stick pan if you can. Try broiling meats. If you fry foods, drain off the extra fat.
- Drain off the oil from canned fish, or buy water-packed fish.
- Make your own low-fat salad dressings. (Recipe on p. 55.)
- Serve low-fat yogurt instead of ice cream.

Eating less salt.

"Why should I eat less salt?"

Too much salt is not good for us.
Most of us eat 3 to 4 times
more salt than we need.

- Too much salt can cause
  high blood pressure.
- Too much salt can make
  you bloated before your
  menstrual periods.
- Too much salt is not good
  for children. If they eat too much salt, they learn
  to like salty foods. This can lead to health
  problems for them when they are older.

"How do I eat less salt?"

- If you want to eat less salt, choose your foods
  carefully. Read the labels on packaged foods.
  You need to avoid ingredients which have **sodium**
  as part of their name. For example, table salt is
  called Sodium Chloride. Many other chemicals
  which are added to your food also contain sodium.
- Even if you don't salt your food, you will have
  to avoid many common foods. There is a lot of
  salt in snack foods, pickles, soy sauce, wieners,
  cold cuts, canned foods, and canned soups. There
  is also a lot of salt in soup mixes, frozen dinners,
  cheese slices, ketchup, and barbecue sauce.

- Avoid processed foods. Processing means changing the food from its natural state. The more processed a food is, the more salt it will contain. Here are some examples:
    - Apple pie contains 100 times more salt than an apple.
    - Fast-food chicken contains 30 times more salt than baked chicken.
    - One frozen TV dinner contains more salt than you need in a whole day.
- Cut down on fast-foods.
- Cut down on salted snack foods, such as chips and crackers.
- Use fewer processed meats such as salami, wieners and bacon.
- Avoid canned soups. They are usually very high in salt. Make your own soups, and use very little salt.
- Take the salt shaker off your table.
- Use garlic and spices to replace the salt you are used to.
- Cut down on canned foods. When you use them, rinse the food under water to get rid of some of the salt.

Eating less sugar.

"Why should I eat less sugar?"

- Too much sugar can make you fat. Foods which contain a lot of sugar have a lot of calories. If you eat too many high-calorie foods you will get fat. People who are fat are more likely to get heart disease and high blood pressure.

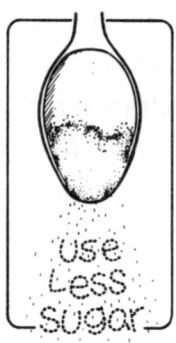

- Too much sugar in your food can lead to tooth decay.

"How do I eat less sugar?"

- If you want to eat less sugar, you will have to choose your foods carefully. You have to start reading the labels on packaged foods. Sugars come in many forms. All the words in this list are sugars: glucose, fructose, sucrose, dextrose, corn syrup, raw sugar, brown sugar, invert sugar, molasses, and honey. Anything which ends in "ose" is a sugar.

Many products have a long list of ingredients. These ingredients are listed in order of amount, starting with the largest. So, if a box of cereal says "sugar, rolled oats, wheat...", then there is more sugar than anything else in this food.

Most of the sugar we eat is hidden in the food we buy. It is in ketchup, canned fruits, soups, pickles, cereals, as well as in cookies, donuts, candies and pop.

- Avoid sweetened cereals. Some of them are almost half sugar. The unsweetened ones are better for you and much cheaper.
- Avoid sweetened canned fruits and fruit juices. Most fresh fruit doesn't need sugar.
- Don't teach your kids to have a sweet tooth. Don't reward them with sweets.
- Cut down on the amount of sugar you use in muffins and cakes. Don't bother with icing.
- Make your own popsicles with fruit juice, or with a mixture of fruit juice and yogurt.
- Some people avoid sugar by eating artificial sweeteners. The sweetener called "aspartame" has become very popular. Aspartame is sold as "NutraSweet and "Equal". Aspartame is added to sugar-free gum, candy, and diet pop. It is also added to fruit drinks, cereal, yogurt, jello desserts, puddings, ice cream bars, cookies, and even vitamin pills.

Aspartame has been tested for safety many times. Scientists think that it is safe, as long as people don't use too much of it. However, no one knows yet how it will effect people who eat it for many years.

The government has decided how much aspartame is safe for children. Now that aspartame is in so many foods, many children eat much more than this amount. This may not be good for them. Until we know more, don't give your children large amounts of aspartame. Until we know more, there is no good reason for pregnant women to eat it at all.

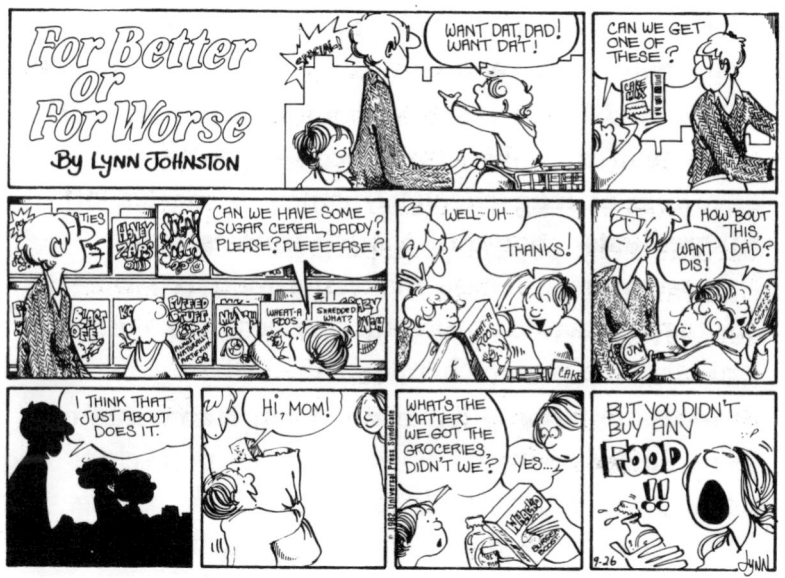

FOR BETTER OR FOR WORSE
COPYRIGHT 1982 UNIVERSAL PRESS SYNDICATE
Reprinted with permission. All rights reserved.

Eating fewer processed foods.

"Why should I cut down on processed food?"

Processed foods are foods which are changed from their natural state. We all eat some processed foods. It is almost impossible to eat only fresh foods. However, we should eat more fresh foods and fewer processed foods. Here's why:

- Processed foods are usually much more expensive than fresh foods. Think about frozen pizza, for example. It has to be prepared, cooked, packaged, stored, delivered, and then stored again. Each of these steps costs money, and you are the one who pays for them.

- Processed foods contain chemical additives. If you read the labels on processed foods, you will see lots of long chemical names in the list of ingredients. Some of these additives are preservatives. These make the food last longer. Some are artificial flavours and colours. A good rule is: the fewer chemicals the better.

- Processed foods often contain large amounts of salt, fat and sugar. Foods such as pop, chips and candy are called "junk food" by many people. This is because they contain so much salt, sugar, fat and chemicals - and not much else.

Cutting down on processed foods will help both your health and your budget.

"How do I cut down on processed foods?"

- Make more of your own foods. It is not hard to make your own salad dressing, spaghetti sauce, or crumb coating for meats. (See recipes from p. 50 to p. 57.)

- Read the labels. Choose foods which are low in sugar, salt, fat and chemicals.

- Cut down on processed meats, such as bacon and salami.

- Avoid junk foods, like chips and donuts.

- Beware of TV ads. Ads put a lot of pressure on us and our children to buy foods, such as chips and sweetened, coloured cereals. Remember: many of these ads tell us things that aren't true. They tell us that candy is a healthy snack. They tell us that athletes depend on candy bars and pop for their strength. This isn't true, but children will believe it unless we tell them that it isn't so.

- The companies who make junk food want to teach you and your children bad eating habits. Don't let them. These companies are interested in one thing - making money. They are not worried about your health, or your children's dental bills. They are not worried about whether or not you will run out of money before pay day. Make up your own mind about what to buy.

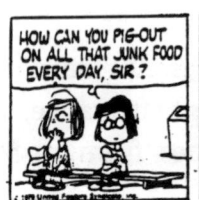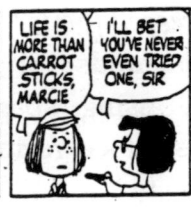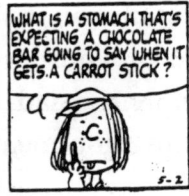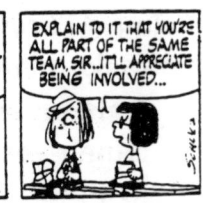

"I'd love to buy good food for my kids but it's so expensive! How can I save money on grocery bills?"

How to save money on your grocery bills.

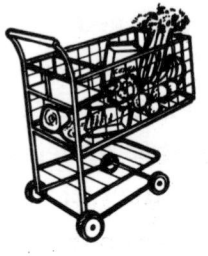

It's hard to make a small income stretch to afford all the foods you need. However, here are some shopping ideas which can help you save money.

- Plan your shopping trips.
  Make a list of what you need to buy. Plan to buy the basics first. Then buy the treats only if you have extra money. Read the ads in the newspaper. Plan some of your meals based on what meats or vegetables are on sale. But, beware. "Bargains" are not always real savings.

- Compare prices.
  - Corner "convenience" stores are usually much more expensive than larger stores.
  - In the larger stores, look for what's cheap. Often the most expensive products are placed at "eye level" so you will pick them first.
  - Check the grade of the food. There is no health difference between Fancy, Choice and Standard. The more expensive ones are just better looking.
  - No-name and store brands are usually cheaper than big-name brands.
  - Larger packages are usually cheaper, but not always. Check for the unit price on the shelf price marker, and choose the cheapest.
- Shop alone if you can. If you must take your children, go at a time when you and your children are not hungry. If you are hungry, you may give in and buy things you don't need.
- Buy in bulk. Fancy wrapping and packaging costs you money. Bulk food stores, some natural food stores, and some grocery stores carry foods in bulk. You can save money on buying flour, noodles, rice, cheese, raisins, nuts, powdered milk, spices, and other foods in bulk.

- **Read the labels.**
  - Many products have a long list of ingredients on the label. These ingredients are listed in order of amount, starting with the largest. So, if a box of cereal says "sugar, rolled oats, wheat...", then you know there is more sugar than any other food in this cereal. The list of ingredients will tell you what you are buying.
  - When you buy packaged food, read the "best before" date to be sure you are getting fresh food.
  - Beware: foods labelled "natural" are not always good for you. They may be high in fat and sugars. Check the list of ingredients.
- **Avoid "convenience foods ".**
  Convenience foods are foods such as packaged pizzas, canned chili, and canned macaroni. They cost a lot. Many packaged foods can be made easily and cheaply at home. (Please see recipes at the end of this chapter.)

"What about cooking? How can I save money cooking?"

How to save money cooking.

Here are some ways to
save money on cooking,
and keep the value in
your food.

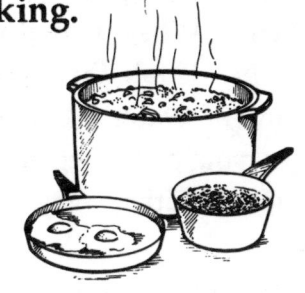

- Avoid using your
  oven too much. The more you use your oven,
  the more electricity or gas you have to pay for.
  Cooking on top of the stove or with appliances is
  cheaper than using your oven. When you do use
  your oven, plan the meal so that the rest of the
  dinner is cooked in the oven too.

- Cook meat at low temperatures, whether you are
  cooking in the oven or on top. This keeps more
  juice in the meat, so it stays moist. It also costs
  you less in hydro.

- Buy cheaper cuts of meat, and cook them slowly
  in liquid. This makes them tender and adds
  flavour. Marinating cheaper cuts of meat before
  cooking has the same effect. Marinating means
  soaking the meat in a liquid such as tomato juice,
  lemon juice, vinegar, wine or beer.

- **Serve raw vegetables** whenever you can. This is because cooking destroys some of the Vitamin C in them. When you do cook vegetables, do it carefully. Cook them for a short time in a small amount of water. Or, better, steam them. The longer you cook vegetables, the more vitamins you lose. Either way, save the water for soup or gravy.
- **Don't soak vegetables.** Don't prepare your vegetables early and soak them in water. Vitamin C is lost into the water.
- **Make soup stock** out of leftover bones. Add a little vinegar to the water. It helps to get the calcium out of the bones and into the stock.
- **Use leftover vegetable cooking water in soups and stews.** Use wilted or fresh vegetables, in soups or stews. Add cooked beans to your soups and stews for extra protein.
- **Uncooked food makes good meals too.** You don't have to cook to make a good meal. There are some healthy fast foods. Whole wheat bread with cheese or peanut butter, fruit, plus milk or juice make a very good meal now and again.

To save money and be healthy:
 Eat more fruit and vegetables.
 Eat more low-fat milk products.
 Eat more whole grains and breads.
    And,
 Eat less junk food,
       less fat,
       less salt,
       less sugar.
 Eat well and feel good.

Chili

Preparation time: 15 minutes.   Cooking time: 50 minutes.

1 medium onion, chopped
1/2 pound of ground beef (Meat can be left out.)
1 teaspoon of Worchestershire sauce (if you like it)
2 teaspoons of chili powder (or more if you like it hot)
1 teaspoon of oregano
2 teaspoons of brown sugar
1 14-ounce can of kidney beans, OR 1/2 cup of dry kidney
  beans, cooked
1 19-ounce can of tomatoes

1. Start with a large heavy pot. If you are using meat,
   cook it over low heat until some of the fat in it melts.
   If you are not using meat, pour 2 or 3 teaspoons of
   cooking oil into the pot.
2. Add the chopped onion, and continue cooking until it is
   soft. (You can also add minced garlic, chopped green
   pepper, and chopped mushrooms at this time. Add
   them to the onion and cook all these vegetables
   together for about 5 minutes. Then continue with the
   rest of the recipe.)
3. Add the other ingredients.
4. Cover the pot and cook over low heat for 30 minutes.
5. Uncover the pot. Simmer the Chili until it thickens.
6. This makes 4 servings.

Spaghetti Sauce

Preparation time: 15 minutes.   Cooking time: 45 minutes.

1 medium onion, chopped

2 teaspoons of cooking oil

1 28-ounce can of tomatoes

1 small can of tomato paste

1 cup of chopped mushrooms (if you like)

1/2 cup of water

1/2 pound of ground beef (or 3/4 cup of Textured
Vegetable Protein. Buy this in a health food store.)

Spices

2 teaspoons of crushed oregano

2 teaspoons of crushed basil

2 small bay leaves

1/2 teaspoon of garlic powder, OR

2 chopped cloves of fresh garlic

1 teaspoon of sugar

1/2 teaspoon of salt

　pepper

1. Use a large saucepan. Cook the onions slowly in the oil
   until they are soft.
2. Add the other ingredients, except the meat or the
   vegetable protein. Cover and cook over low heat for
   15 minutes.
3. Add the meat or the vegetable protein. Stir, cover, and
   cook over low heat for another 30 minutes.
4. Remove the bay leaves.
5. Serve with spaghetti, lasagna, or on pizza.
6. This makes 4 to 6 servings. It freezes well.

Crispy Crumb Coating Oven Mix

Preparation time: 5 minutes

2 cups of dry bread crumbs
1/4 cup of vegetable oil
1 teaspoon of salt
a couple shakes of pepper
1 1/2 teaspoon of paprika
1 teaspoon of poultry seasoning, OR
   1 teaspoon of a mixture of sage and thyme
1/4 teaspoon of garlic powder, or more if you wish

1. Mix the ingredients well. Now the Oven Mix is ready to use.
2. Preheat the oven to 350 °F. Put some of the Oven Mix in a bag. Remove the skin from the chicken pieces, and then moisten them with milk or water. Drop each piece into the bag, and then shake it until the meat is coated with Mix.
3. Lay the chicken in a shallow pan in the oven. Bake for about one hour, or until cooked.
4. Store the extra Mix in a covered container in the fridge.
5. This Mix can also be used with pork, veal, or fish.

Coleslaw

Preparation time: 10 minutes

<u>Dressing</u>:
1/4 cup of sugar
1/4 cup of oil
1/2 cup of vinegar
1/2 teaspoon of salt
1/2 teaspoon of dry mustard
1/2 teaspoon of ground celery seed
   pepper
Mix the dressing ingredients together in a small saucepan. Bring it to a boil. Let it cool.

<u>Vegetables</u>:
1 small cabbage, thinly sliced or grated
1/2 thinly sliced onion
1 medium carrot, grated

1. Mix the cabbage, onion, and carrot together.
2. Pour the dressing over the vegetables. Stir well.
3. Cover and store the salad in the fridge.

Fruit Cabbage Salad

Preparation time: 10 minutes

Dressing:
1/2 cup of plain yogurt
1/2 cup of mayonnaise
1 teaspoon of grated lemon rind
1 or 2 teaspoons of orange juice
1 teaspoon of sugar

Mix the dressing ingredients together.

Vegetables:
1 small head cabbage, shredded
2 or 3 apples, chopped (OR use both apples and pears)
1/2 cup raisins
1/4 cup of nuts, chopped
1 teaspoon of lemon juice

1. Combine cabbage with fruit and nuts and lemon juice.
2. Pour dressing over salad and mix well. Chill in fridge.

Thousand Island Dressing

Preparation time: 5 minutes

1 cup of light mayonnaise
1/4 cup of ketchup
1 tablespoon of chopped onion
3 tablespoons of relish (OR 2 small pickles, chopped)
2 tablespoons of chopped green pepper (if you like)

Mix all the ingredients together in a jar.   Store in fridge.

(Dressing can also be made using 1/2 cup light
mayonnaise and 1/2 cup of plain yogurt, instead of
1 cup of mayonnaise.)

Dip for Vegetables

Preparation time: 5 minutes

1 cup of plain yogurt
1 clove of garlic, chopped, OR 1/2 teaspoon of garlic
powder

1. Mix the ingredients in a bowl. Chill the mixture in
   the fridge for about an hour.
2. Other flavours can also be added, such as green
   onions, dill weed, hot chilies, and curry. Try different
   flavours and see what your family likes.
3. Serve with cut-up vegetables such as:

broccoli	green onions
cauliflower	mushrooms
carrots	radishes
celery	snow peas
cucumbers	tomatoes
green beans	turnip
green pepper	zucchini.

4. If you want a richer dip, use
   1 cup of yogurt and 2 tablespoons of mayonnaise, OR
   1/2 cup of yogurt and 1/2 cup of light sour cream.

Bran Muffins

Preparation time: 10 minutes.   Cooking time: 15 minutes

1 cup of vegetable oil

2 cups of sugar

6 eggs

4 tablespoons of molasses

3 cups of milk

5 cups of cooking bran (not prepared cereal)

3 cups of white flour, OR

    2 cups of white flour, plus

    1 cup of whole wheat flour

1 teaspoon of salt

2 teaspoons of baking powder

1 teaspoon of baking soda

1 1/2 cups of cut-up dates or raisins

1. Beat together the oil, sugar, and the eggs.
2. Add the rest of the ingredients and stir. Just mix enough to make the flour disappear.
3. Store the batter in the fridge for a few hours.
4. Preheat the oven to 425°F. Spoon the batter into greased muffin tins and bake for about 15 minutes.
5. This batter can be kept several weeks in a covered container in the fridge.
6. This recipe makes 4 dozen good muffins.

Dealing With Your "Nerves"

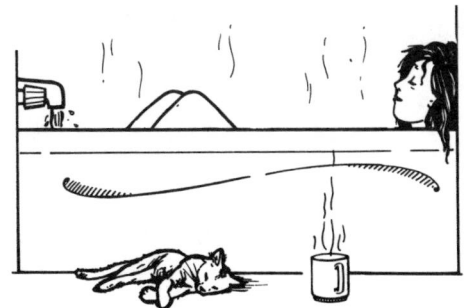

DEALING WITH YOUR "NERVES"

"Bad nerves" and stress.

All of us have trouble with our "nerves" sometimes. When your nerves are bothering you, you may show it in different ways. You may become tense and edgy, or you may have trouble sleeping. You may cry a lot, or you may have stomach troubles. When you talk about your "bad nerves", you are really talking about stress, and how it is affecting you.

Stress is a hard thing to describe because it isn't the same for each person. It affects people in different ways. For example, driving in heavy traffic may give you a headache. However, it may make someone else tense and grouchy.

Stress is also hard to describe because the same event may bother one person and not another. For example, your sister may love having lots of people for dinner, but you may hate it.

Not only is stress different for each person; it won't always be the same for you. You'll be able to handle much more stress some days than others. For example, things may bother you much more when you are tired or before your period. Or, you may notice stress when you have several things to do at once. Even if some of the things are fun, all together, they may be just too much.

Stress itself is not a bad thing. Life would be boring if everything went along smoothly all the time. And, some stress is useful. It can make you learn new things. It can make you try new things. Stress can make you do things you never thought you could do.

However, we all have a limit to how much we can handle. When we go over our limit, then too much stress can be harmful. Whether your stress comes from good things or bad things, too much stress will affect you. It will affect how you feel, and how you act.

"How do I know if I'm under too much stress?"

If you are under too much stress, you may notice that you feel different. Most of us have some warning signs which tell us that we are near our limit. Learn to notice what yours are. Learn to pay attention to them.

Warning signs of too much stress.

1. Too much stress can affect how you feel.
   - You may be jumpy or on edge.
   - You may be weepy.
   - You may be bad tempered.
   - You may be very critical of yourself.
   - You may be very critical of people you used to like.

2. Too much stress can affect how you act.
   - You may smoke more.
   - You may drink more alcohol.
   - You may eat much more (or much less).
   - You may be less able to do things which used to be easy.

3. Too much stress can affect your body.
   - You may have tense, sore muscles in your neck, jaw or back.
   - You may have headaches.
   - You may have stomach problems.
   - You may have sleeping problems.
   - You may have skin rashes.
   - You may have changes in your menstrual periods.
   - You may be sick much more than usual.
   - You may be tired all the time.

These are a few common signs of too much stress. You may have different signs, or none at all.

Health problems from stress.

Too much stress for too long can make you sick. At first, you may get more colds or flu. If you are under stress for too long, you may also get:
- migraine headaches
- ulcers
- high blood pressure
- heart disease.

Too much stress can also lead to depression. If you want to know more about depression, you could read Chapter 3, <u>Depression</u>.

Even though stress doesn't always make you sick, you use up a lot of energy dealing with it. Too much stress can make you feel very tired. It can make you less able to deal with new things as they come along. That's why it's so important to control stress before it controls you.

Dealing with stress.

If you feel a lot of stress, you may have a lot to cope with. You already have some good ways of coping with stress. It might help to learn some more ways as well. "Bad nerves" shouldn't be a way of life. You can change some things and you can feel much better.

To deal with stress:
Step One: Figure out what the cause is.
Step Two: Make some changes in your life.
Step Three: Take good care of yourself.

Step One: Figure out what the cause is.
When you notice that you have too much stress, you need to figure out what is bothering you. We are all different, so different things bother different people. Even so, some things cause stress for most people.

Here are some common sources of stress. Read through the lists, and see if any of these things bother you.

1. Big changes often cause stress.

Big changes in your lives are often sources of stress. Even if they happened long ago, they may still affect you.

Here are some big changes:
- the birth of a new baby
- the death of a relative or friend
- marriage
- divorce or separation
- retirement
- the loss of your job or your partner's job
- return to work after many years
- a move to a new town
- a serious sickness
- a new person to look after, such as an aging parent.

Remember: even events which you look forward to, such as a birth or a wedding, can be hard on you.

2. Everyday problems often cause stress.

Everyday problems cause stress for everyone. Some problems are more serious than others, but they can all get us down.

Here are some common everyday problems which can cause stress:

- Having arguments or fights with your partner or your husband, or with your children, your neighbours, or your boss.
- Not having enough money. Without money, it's very hard to be in control of the important things in your life. Without money, you don't have as much power to do what you want to do. You may not be able to go back to school, or to move, or to buy enough fresh foods. You may not be able to buy all the things your children need.
- Having too many jobs and too many things you are responsible for - and not enough help.

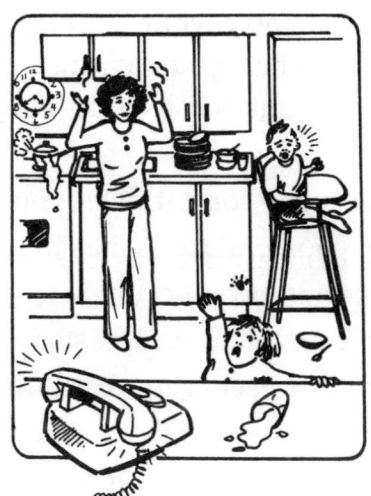

- Having health problems or injuries.
- Being bored from too little to do, or from having too many boring jobs to do.
- Having less control in your family or at your job because you are a woman.

- Having an unpleasant job that is dangerous or low paying.
- Having too many people around, or having no one around when you need them.
- Always rushing; to get to work, to get your kids to school, to get supper made.

3. Worrying often causes stress.

Worrying about things that might happen can cause stress. Many people bring extra stress on themselves by worrying too much. It makes sense to be concerned about some things, but **worrying by itself won't solve your problems.** Worrying can wear you out. Then you may not have any energy left to figure out what to do about your problem.

Here are some things you may be worried about:
- your children's health
- your own health
- your children's custody
- your teenagers' behaviour
- your marriage or your relationship
- your safety at home or at work
- your husband's bad temper.

You may also be worried about:
- being able to afford what you need
- finding a better job
- paying your bills
- finding a better place to live
- taking care of your parents or relatives
- growing old.

If you are worried, try to figure out what is bothering you. Try to figure out what you can do about your problem. For example, if you are worried about your health, go to the doctor, and find out more. Or, if you think you need help with your relationship, find a counsellor and get some help. Or, if you are worried about money, get credit counselling.

Don't wear yourself out worrying. Save some energy to solve your problems.

4. Your reactions often cause stress.

You can make problems for yourself by how you react to things that happen.

This may be a new idea for you. You may think that only events make you upset, not how you respond to them. However, how you react can make things worse.

For example, the bus driver was rude to both you and your friend. You just laughed it off, but your friend was angry and upset about it for a long time. She felt bad because she took the bus driver's comments personally. A lot of the stress she felt came from how she reacted. She would have had less stress if she had not let herself get so upset.

5. Things which you cannot control often cause stress.

All your stress does not come from the way you handle your problems. Some of it comes from the world we live in. We all feel stress from things which we cannot control.

Problems like poverty, wife beating, rape, child abuse, nuclear war, and pollution affect us all. These problems bring stress because they are so difficult to solve, especially all alone. However, there are some things you can do. You can work together with other women to make this a safer world.

For example, if you were raped, you could get together with other women who were raped. You could give each other support, and you could work on making your apartment building safer.

You could also join a tenant's group or an anti-nuclear group. Or, you could help out in a women's shelter or in an after-school program. These are just a few examples of the ways women can work together to make changes.

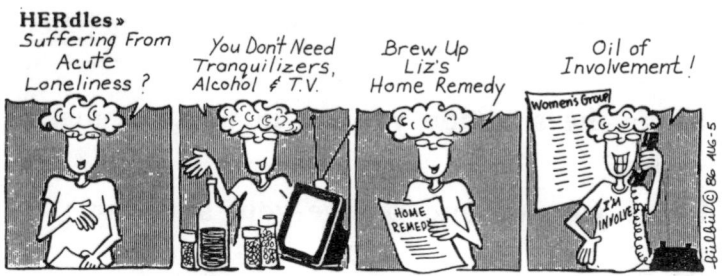

© Bulbul, 1986

After you know what is causing your stress, you need to figure out what to do about it. The next section talks about how to deal with some of the causes of stress which you can change yourself.

To deal with stress:
Step One: Figure out what the cause is.
Step Two: Make some changes in your life.
Step Three: Take good care of yourself.

Step Two: Make some changes in your life.

When you have a lot of stress, it means that something has to change.

You have three choices:
1. **Change yourself** so that things don't bother you as much.
2. **Change the situation** you are in which is making you upset.
3. **Change yourself and change your situation.**

Some people use this AA (Alcoholics Anonymous) prayer to help them decide what to change:

"Grant me
the serenity to accept the things I cannot change,
the courage to change the things I can, and
the wisdom to know the difference."

Here are some ideas for how to start changing parts of your life. Remember: make your changes one step at a time. Don't try too much at once, or you may create more problems.

(1) You can change things by being more assertive.

You can get rid of some of the stress in your life by being more assertive. Being assertive doesn't mean being selfish or pushy. It doesn't mean being cruel, or trying to get even. Being assertive means saying what you want and what you think. It means believing that you have as much right to get what you need as anyone else does. It means standing up for what you want, and taking some control over what happens to you.

Being assertive can be hard for women. Many of us were raised to be good girls. We were taught to be very obedient. We were taught to always take care of our family before ourselves. There is nothing wrong with taking care of others. However, if we don't also take care of ourselves sometimes, we may never get what we need.

If you are interested, you could take an "Assertiveness Course for Women". Many community colleges and YWCAs offer these courses.

(2) You can change things by removing some of the sources of stress.

You can get rid of some stress by removing some of the things which are problems for you.

- You may have trouble with your marriage. You and your partner may fight a lot. You may be afraid of him. He may put you down a lot, and he may hurt you.

If you are having problems with your partner or your children, be sure to get some outside help. Even if your partner won't go with you, go for help yourself. An outside person is often very useful.

If you want to, call and talk with a counsellor at a shelter for battered women. If you are in any danger, you can go to a shelter. You will be safe there while you decide what to do next.

In Ontario, women's shelters are listed under "W" in the white pages as Wife Assault Helpline. Sometimes shelters are also listed on the front page of the phone book. If you can't find the number, you could get the number from a Crisis Centre, a Distress Centre, an Information Centre, or the police. Their numbers are usually on the front page of the phone book.

- You may have friends or family that you don't get along with. Perhaps, you could see them less often.
- You may have a job which you hate. You might be able to talk things over with your boss, or maybe you could change jobs. Your job might be better if you belonged to a union.
- You may never get time alone. There may be times when someone else could take care of your children. You could trade babysitting with a friend. You could watch your friend's children one morning, and she could watch yours the next day.
- You may be lonely. You could join a single parents' group, or a women's group, or a widow's group.
- You may have chores which you hate. You could drop them. For example, maybe you could stop sending Christmas cards. Or, maybe you could not wash the floor so often, or not iron so often, or not make dessert for every meal. Maybe you could get your partner or your children to give you more help with the chores.

Remember: You can always make more changes than you think.

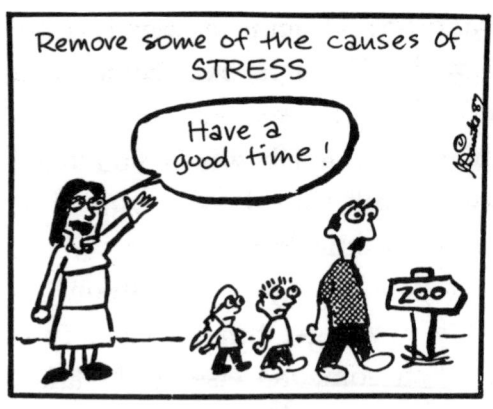

(3) You can change things by changing how you react to problems.

Some of us have a bad habit. We react to upsetting things in ways that make us more upset.

If you often feel angry, or jealous, or hurt, or suspicious, ask yourself these questions:
- Do I know enough about what happened to feel this way?
- Do my feelings help me figure out what happened?
- Do my feelings help me figure out what should be done?
- Do my feelings make me feel better or worse?
- Could I react in a different way that would be easier on me?

You may find that your reactions make you more upset than you need to be. Before you get upset, make sure that you are not taking the wrong meaning from things before you have all the facts. If you can stop yourself from getting too easily upset, you will feel less stress.

I am not saying that you should never get upset. I am not saying that you should just accept unfair things in your life. But, if you change how you react, you will leave yourself enough energy to work on whatever needs changing.

Some people handle some of their stress by looking for the funny side of things. This way of reacting to problems helps them get through tough times. Healthy people know how to laugh at themselves. Laughing at yourself and the world around you means you can accept your mistakes and still carry on. Learning to laugh at things is a good way to get rid of some stress.

When things are getting you down, watch a funny TV show or a funny movie. You'll be surprised how much better you will feel. Doctors know that laughing is useful. Some hospitals have programs to try to make their patients laugh because it helps them get better! Laughing is good for you. "Laughter really is the best medicine".

Even if you have serious problems, don't feel guilty if you take some time out to enjoy yourself. It will help you cope.

(4) You can change things by changing how you talk to yourself.

Many of us talk to ourselves. And when we do, we tell ourselves things which make us feel bad! This way, we make more problems for ourselves than the ones we already have.

For example, when we do something wrong, we say things like: *"I'm so stupid. I can't do anything right! I was always so stupid (or clumsy, or silly, or lazy, or helpless, or ...)."*

These are called put-downs. Our parents or teachers may have said these things to us when we were young. Our partners or friends may say these things to us now. Sometimes they say these things seriously. Sometimes they say them as jokes. However, the message is still there.

If we hear these put-downs often enough, we begin to believe them. Then we start saying them to ourselves too. When we make mistakes, we go on putting ourselves down.

Not only do put-downs make us feel bad. They are also unrealistic. That is, they don't give us a true picture of what is going on. No one is always stupid or lazy or helpless or anything else. We are all stupid or lazy or helpless sometimes. And, we are all clever and full of energy and able to do a lot at other times. Put-downs like these prevent us from seeing what we are really like.

Although it is hard work, you can change the things you say to yourself. When you make a mistake, don't tell yourself what a dummy you are. Instead, say something like: *"Sure I made a mistake. Everyone makes mistakes sometimes. It doesn't mean I'm stupid. No one is perfect."*

Next time things go wrong, listen to what you are telling yourself. Check to see if you are making things worse by telling yourself unrealistic things. See if you are expecting unrealistic things of yourself. If you are, then you may be making it harder for yourself to cope.

Below is a list of some of the unrealistic and harmful things we often tell ourselves. Each one is followed by a more realistic and useful way of looking at things. Read through the list, and see if any of them are like the things you say to yourself.

Stop saying this: I have always been like this, and I will be like this for the rest of my life.

✔ Start saying this: I have changed in lots of ways. I will go on changing and learning things all through my life.

Stop saying this: I need someone strong to depend on.

✔ Start saying this: I am a strong woman and I've made it this far. We all need help and support sometimes. That doesn't mean that we are weak. In the end, I can still depend on me.

Stop saying this: I am going to fail, I know it.

✔ Start saying this: I've been through tough times before, and I came through. I can handle this.

Stop saying this: If I say what I want, people will get mad at me and hurt me. I must never upset other people.

✔ Start saying this: I have the right to ask for what I want. If I do, some people may respect me, and some may help me. Some people may also be angry with me. If they don't like it, that's their problem. I can't change them.

If I say what I want, things often get better. If it is dangerous for me to say what I want, then I need to change my life so that I will be safe.

Stop saying this: Of course I am unhappy; look at all the bad things that have happened to me.

✔ Start saying this: Bad things that happen do affect me. However, I still have some control over how I react to them. I can react in ways which won't make me more upset.

Stop saying this: When something goes wrong between me and someone else, it must be my fault.

✔ Start saying this: When things go wrong, it may be because of something I did, but it may not be. I will stop blaming myself for everything which goes wrong. Feeling guilty about the past doesn't help anything.

Stop saying this: If I keep worrying then maybe bad things won't happen.

✔ Start saying this: My worrying only makes me unhappy and tense. Worrying about the future doesn't help anything. I won't go around being afraid and saying "What if?".

Stop saying this: I must be perfect and not make any mistakes. If I make mistakes, people will know that I am stupid. If I ask for help, people will know that I am weak. If I don't try anything new, then I won't make many mistakes.

✓ **Start saying this:** I don't have to be perfect, and I'm not. Everyone makes mistakes. I can learn from my mistakes. If I try something new, I'll learn something new.

If I need help I will ask for it. We all need help sometimes. No one is perfect.

I am a valuable person no matter how well I do things. I won't compare myself to others anymore.

Stop saying this: So-and-so doesn't like me; this is awful!

✓ **Start saying this:** Not everyone will like me. I don't need to be upset if one person doesn't like me, or doesn't agree with me.

Stop saying this: I must help other people solve their problems.

✔ **Start saying this:** I can choose if I want to help other people with their problems. When people ask for help, I can say "yes" or "no". I have important needs too.

Next time you feel bad, think about what you are saying to yourself. Change how you talk to yourself, and you can make yourself feel better.

(5) You can change things by getting organized.

A good way to cut down on stress is to get organized. Well-organized people don't depend on their memory. They write everything down.

If you have trouble remembering things, get yourself two calendars. Get a big one for your wall, and a little one for your purse. You can get calendars free from some banks and stores around the new year, or you can make your own.

Then write down everything which you need to remember. Write down every appointment, every important day at your kids' school, and any other dates you need to remember. Write down any important thing you have to do every month, such as paying the rent, or checking on your budget. Some people use words, and some people use pictures. Some people use special colours to remind them of special things. Try to find a way that works well for you.

If you have every important thing written down, you won't have to worry about forgetting things. You also won't have the stress of having to make new arrangements after you forget.

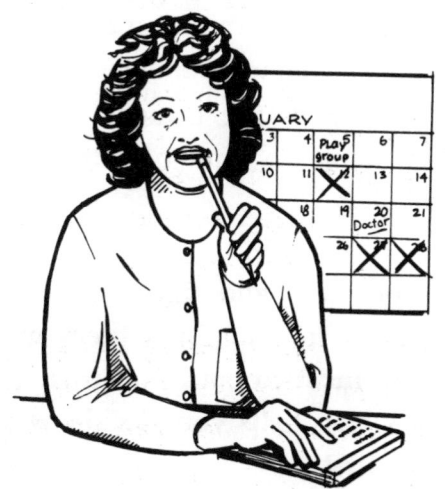

If you write things down and keep a few lists, you might feel more in control. You can make lists of the things which you have to do the next day. You can make lists for shopping, for Christmas ideas, and for free events to take your children to.

Lists will also help you deal with big problems or big jobs. The whole problem or the whole job may seem too big to handle. However, any job is made up of many smaller jobs. If you make a list of the smaller jobs, it will be much easier to know where to start.

If you have a lot to do, it can be hard to know where to start. One way to figure this out is to make two lists.

- Make one list of the things you have to do. These are the kind of things that will make more problems if you don't do them.
- Make another list of the things you would like to do. These are the kind of things that can wait for a while.

Then look at your lists and figure out which jobs are the most important to do. Give them numbers, starting with the most important, down to the least important. This will help you decide which things you need to do first.

Getting organized with calendars and lists will help you deal with your busy life.

(6) You can change things by making a new routine.

You may have a lot of stress because you need a new routine. If you are always behind, you may need a new time-table. For example, you might need to get your children up fifteen minutes earlier in the morning. This would give you enough time to eat and get to work without rushing.

You may need to change your routine to make time for a few breaks during the day. If you forget, set an alarm. You may also need to make time to unwind before bed.

Some people who are really busy plan their day carefully. First they do the things they hate most. Then they don't have unpleasant jobs hanging over them all day long. They also save the nice jobs for later on in the day. Then their day gets better as it goes along. Other people do an unpleasant job first, then a nice one, then an unpleasant one, and so on.

Try some different ways to change your routine until you find a way that is best for you.

To deal with stress:

Step One: Figure out what the cause is.

Step Two: Make some changes in your life.

Step Three: Take good care of yourself.

Step Three: Take good care of yourself.

Last but not least, you need to take good care of yourself. Taking care of yourself is important all the time. However, it is really important when you are under a lot of stress.

No one can avoid stress completely. But, if you take good care of yourself, stress won't be as hard on you. You will be able to deal with problems as they come along, so things won't get worse. If you feel good, you will be able to make changes much more easily.

(1) Take good care of yourself by taking good care of your body.

When you are under stress, it is very important to remember to take good care of your body. You use up a lot of energy dealing with stress. You can replace some of this energy by exercising, by eating well, and by avoiding drugs and alcohol.

Here are some ways to cut down on the "wear and tear" on your body due to stress:

• **Be more active.** Exercise is a great way to let off steam. Exercise helps you get rid of tension in your muscles. It also helps you to sleep better. Even a ten minute walk can make you feel much better. If you want more information on ways to be more active, please read Chapter 4, <u>Being Active</u>.

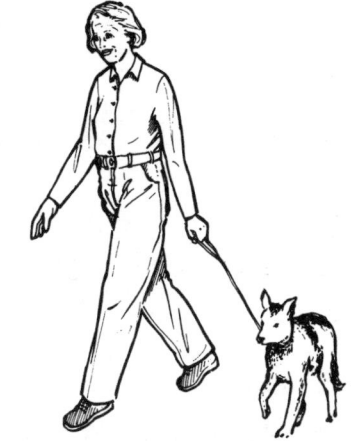

• **Eat healthy, regular meals.** Eat good meals, even if you don't feel like it. Don't expect your body to feel good on cigarettes and coffee alone.

If you want more information on food for "People with Bad Nerves", please read p. 31 in Chapter 1, <u>Eating Well</u>.

• **Don't depend on pills.** Tranquillizers and sedatives, such as Valium and Ativan, are not the harmless drugs many people think they are.

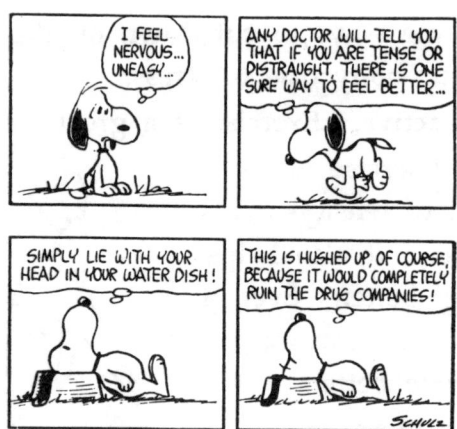

© 1967 United Feature Syndicate, Inc.

Tranquillizers don't solve problems. They don't teach you new ways to cope. They can make you drowsy, depressed, and less able to think clearly. If you take them for a long time, you may be less able to figure out your problems. You may feel too tired and confused to think straight.

There is another problem with taking tranquillizers for a long time. You can become addicted to them. Then it can become very hard to stop taking them.

Tranquillizers can also be very dangerous if you take them along with alcohol. This is because both alcohol and tranquillizers affect your brain in the same way. Together they make you very drowsy. Too much of them together can even kill you.

If you and your doctor think that you really need tranquillizers, take them for only a couple weeks at a time.

If you have been taking them for a long time and you want to stop, get some advice. Talk with an addictions counsellor or a doctor, and stop taking them gradually. Don't stop all at once or you may feel terrible.

• **Cut down on cigarettes, coffee and alcohol.**

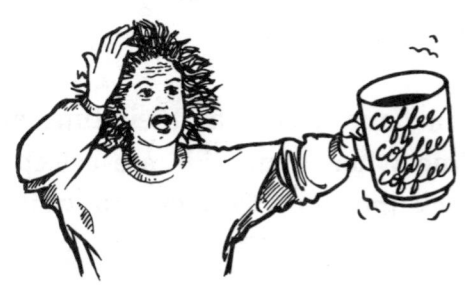

Many people smoke a lot and drink a lot of coffee when their nerves are bad. This is a mistake. These things will just make you more jittery in the long run. They also prevent you from sleeping well. Without sleep, no one can cope well for very long. Many people drink more when they are upset. Drinking is never a good way to deal with your problems. Alcohol is hard on your body. You can also get addicted to it.

If you think you may have a drinking problem, be sure to get help. You could get help from AA, or from an addictions counsellor, or from your public health nurse. The sooner you get help, the easier it is to quit.

(2) Take good care of yourself by making some time for yourself.

Every day you need some time just for you. Time-just-for-you is not time for housework or shopping. It is time to do whatever you please. When you are very busy, remind yourself that you deserve some time to relax and daydream.

Many women have a bath as their time alone. Choose a time when your kids are asleep or at school, or lock the door to keep out visitors.

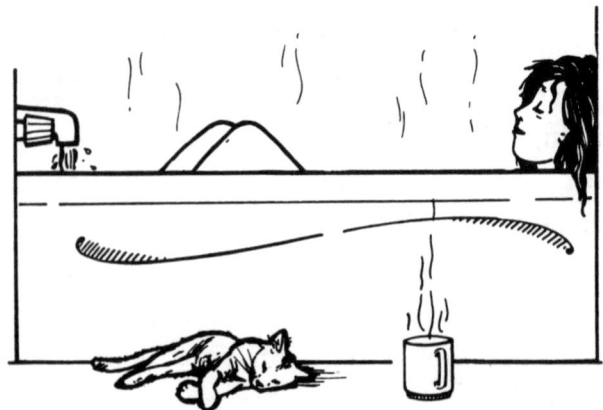

Some women go for walks. Others do hobbies such as jigsaw puzzles and knitting. Others just sit with their feet up. Others read, and others meditate. Some women like to do things outside their home. Some like bingo, sports, church work, and visiting friends. Others enjoy doing volunteer work.

Even if you can only manage a couple of 5 minute breaks in a day, take them and enjoy them. Close your eyes and breathe deeply for 5 minutes and you will feel better.

Women with small children really need regular breaks. If you have children at home all day, it won't be easy to get time for yourself. One way is to trade babysitting with a friend. And remember; kids are only young for a short time. You won't be stuck at home forever.

Whatever you enjoy doing, try to make some time every day to do what you want to do. Learn to make time just for you.

(3) Take good care of yourself by getting help and support.

Everyone has trouble coping sometimes. When you have a problem, don't try to cope all alone. Don't keep all your problems bottled up inside. One of the best things to do for yourself is to talk with a friend, or someone in your family, or a counsellor.

Talking - or laughing or crying - will help you to think more clearly. Sympathy and support from a friend will cut down on your stress. If you talk over your problems with a friend, then you won't be carrying all your problems alone.

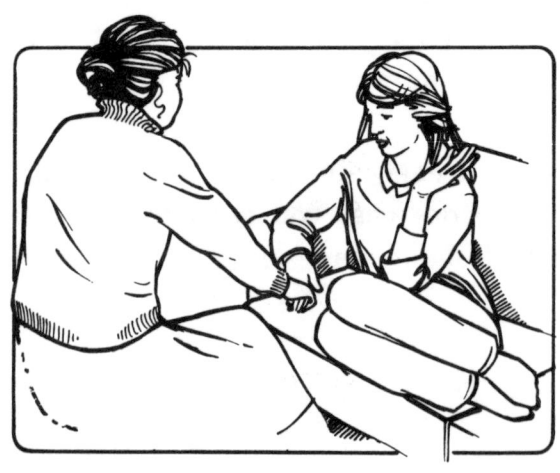

There are many people who are trained to help people to deal with stress. The Information Bureau in your town can help you find a good counsellor whom you can afford. And, if you are not happy with your counsellor, keep looking until you find someone you like.

You could also join a **support group**. In a support group you could talk with other people who are in a situation like yours.

For example, you could join a group for mothers of small children. There you could talk with other mothers about the fun and hassles of raising children. You might get some ideas about ways to deal with problems, such as coping with a sick child. You could also have the fun of talking with other adults while your children play with other children.

There are many different kinds of support groups. There are some for single parents, and some for people with health and emotional problems. If you want to know about the groups in your community, call the Information Bureau, or your Health Unit, or your local women's centre.

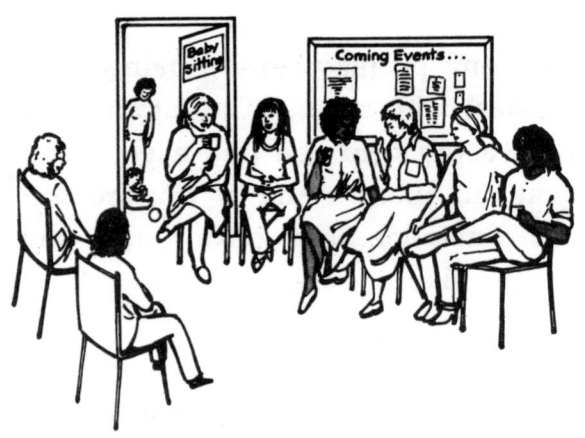

If a group doesn't exist, you could start your own. You don't need to be an expert to start a group. Most of these groups were begun by people like you — people who had a problem, and who wanted to talk to others "in the same boat".

(4) Take good care of yourself by not expecting too much of yourself.

If you have had a large change in your life, you may need time to get used to it. Don't expect yourself to adjust right away.

Even if you were looking forward to something, such as a marriage or a new baby, you may need time to adjust. Or if a friend dies, you will need time to get used to loosing that person from your life. This time is called an "adjustment period", and it is something which you have to go through.

While you are adjusting, take good care of yourself. And make sure that you tell yourself how well you are coping, even if no one else does.

If you have several problems to deal with at once, don't be too hard on yourself. Don't expect yourself to cope perfectly. Take one problem at a time. Start with something easy.

Many women expect too much of themselves. They think that they should be a wife, and a mother, and a working woman without any problems. Then they are upset when they find out they are only human.

Check to see if you are expecting more of yourself than any one woman could do. Letting yourself be human is a good way to start taking good care of yourself.

If you want an end to your "bad nerves", remember these ideas:

1. **Watch for the warning signs of too much stress.**

You might be on edge or you might cry more easily. You might be smoking, or drinking, or eating more. You might have more headaches, or tense, sore muscles. You might have stomach problems or sleeping problems. You might notice that you are sick more than usual, or that you are tired all the time.

2. **Figure out what is bothering you.**

Is it a big thing, or a lot of small things, or both?

3. **Make some changes.**

Figure out what has to change, and then change what you can.

4. **Take good care of yourself.**

Take good care of your health, and be sure to get support from your friends.

5. **Keep your sense of humour.**

Depression

3

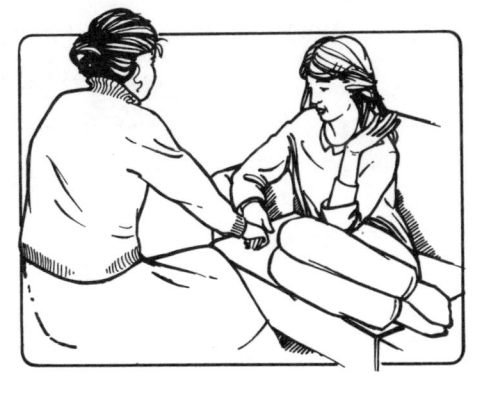

DEPRESSION

There are two different kinds of depression:
1. Short Depression.

This is the kind of depression which we all feel now and again when we are down in the dumps. This kind of depression usually doesn't last very long.

2. Long-Lasting Depression.

This is a much more serious kind of depression. This depression is like a terrible, endless sadness. This kind of depression usually lasts quite a while. When people have this kind of depression, they may not even realize it. They may not say they are depressed. Instead, they may say that nothing much matters any more.

If you are depressed, it is important to know what kind of depression you have. If you are just feeling down, you can usually help yourself. You can usually start feeling better if you take better care of yourself, and if you work on your problems. You usually will not need help from a therapist. However, if you have a serious, long-lasting depression, you will likely need some help from a therapist or a counsellor.

The first part of this chapter talks about the feelings of depression which we all have once in a while. In this part you can read about some of the reasons you may feel down. You can also read about some ways to make yourself feel better. The second part talks about serious, long-lasting depressions. You can read about some reasons these depressions happen, and what you can do about them.

1. Common short depressions.

"I'm really bummed out today."

Many things can make you feel down for a while:

- You may feel sad and depressed for a time after you hear some bad news.
- You may feel down and discouraged if you have problems with your husband or your partner.
- You may feel depressed when you are swamped with work.
- You may feel depressed for a while if you are at home with young children during bad weather.
- You may feel down around Christmas time.
- You may feel sad around the anniversary of a loved one's death.
- You may feel depressed for a few days before your period every month.

These are the ups and downs of normal life. We all go through times like this.

Coping when you feel down.

Here are some ways to help you feel better.

1. Start moving.

Being active helps you feel better, in your body and in your mind. The more you move, the better you'll feel. People who exercise regularly are more able to deal with day-to-day problems. Some people find that just a 15 minute walk every day makes them feel much better.

Before you start, you may really not feel like doing anything, but afterwards you will feel much better. If you make yourself get some exercise every day - even for just a little while - you will feel better, and you will sleep better.

(If you want more informaion about being active, please read Chapter 4, Getting Fit.)

2. Eat well.

Eat at least 2 good meals a day, whether you feel like it or not. If you don't eat, you'll feel even worse. If you want to know more about eating well, please read Chapter 1, Eating Well.

3. Cut down on how much alcohol you drink.

Alcohol is a depressant drug. This means that it can make you feel depressed. You may feel happier after a few drinks. However, after that, the alcohol will make you feel more depressed.

4. Cut down on how much coffee and tea you drink.

Coffee and tea contain caffeine which is a "stimulant". This means that drinking coffee or tea in the evening will make it harder for you to get a good sleep. And, when you are tired, it's much harder to cope with anything.

5. Keep busy.

Don't sit around by yourself too much or you may feel worse. Try to keep busy doing things even though you may not feel like it.

This may sound corny, but a very good way to make yourself feel better is to do something for someone else. Groups such as hospitals, YWCAs, immigrant service groups and schools are always looking for volunteers. We all have something to share with someone else. If you want to be a volunteer, call the Volunteer Bureau in your area.

6. Keep in touch with your friends.

Friends can be good medicine. Keep in touch with your friends and let them take care of you a little. Don't be embarrassed to let them see you down. We all feel bad sometimes.

7. Give yourself a break.

Try to get a break every day. Even short breaks can do wonders. Maybe you could trade baby-sitting with a friend. Ask her to watch your children while you go out, or while you have some time by yourself. Later you could do the same for her.

8. Treat yourself.

We often forget how good little treats can make us feel. Perhaps you could meet a friend and go for an ice cream. Or, you could buy yourself a magazine. Or, you could have a long bath and go to bed really early. Try to remember the things that made you feel good as a child, and try some of them. You know best what would be a treat for you.

9. Don't worry too much.

Many people think that they are solving their problems if they are worrying about them. However, worrying - by itself - doesn't change anything. It just leaves you tired and more depressed. Try not to just worry about your problems. Instead, try to solve them.

10. Try to face your problems.

Trying to avoid your problems for a long time can be more tiring and depressing than working on them! If you need help to deal with your problems, then get help. Talk with a friend about what is bothering you. Problems are often much easier to handle after you have talked them over with someone else.

11. Think carefully about your problems.

Ask yourself:

- Which problems are most important?
- Which problems can I do something about?
- Which ones can I leave for now?
- Who can I talk to about my problems?

When you know the answers to these questions, you will know more about where to begin.

12. Don't let your nerves get the better of you.

If you want to know more about how to deal your "bad nerves", you could read Chapter 2, <u>Dealing With Your "Nerves"</u>.

Next time you feel down in the dumps, try one or two of these ideas for coping. Find out which ones work best for you.

2. Long-lasting serious depressions.

"Nothing seems to make me feel any better."

Besides the short, sad times which we all have now and again, some people become seriously depressed.

If you have never been depressed, it is hard to imagine. It is much worse than feeling down for a few days. It feels more like a terrible sadness that never goes away.

Depression can affect your whole life. It can affect how you feel and how you act. It makes you feel miserable, and then it makes you less able to do anything about it.

Signs of depression.

- You and your friends may say that you are "not yourself anymore".
- You may be less interested in the things you used to enjoy.
- You may not want to see other people.
- You might be less interested in food or sex.
- You may have headaches.
- You may feel sick.
- You may feel very tired, and you may have trouble sleeping.

- You may often wake up very early in the morning. After you wake up, you may not be able to get back to sleep.
- You may have trouble thinking and making decisions.
- You may feel worthless.
- You may say that you are "just existing". You may feel that nothing matters, and nothing seems worth doing.
- You may even think about killing yourself.

Suicide:

Remember, people do kill themselves. Many people think about killing themselves, and many do it. One out of every seven depressed people kills themself. If you have been seriously thinking about suicide, talk to someone about it. You may think that suicide is the only solution to your problems, but it is not. It is not a solution to your problems or to your family's problems. If you had help, you wouldn't feel so bad, and then you wouldn't want to die.

It you know someone who is talking about committing suicide, try to get them some help. Call a Crisis Centre, or a member of their family, or their doctor. Never think that someone won't kill themselves just because they have talked about it before. Always take a threat of suicide seriously.

"Why do I feel like this?"

There are three kinds of serious depressions:
1. Depressions that are caused by health problems.
2. Depressions that are caused by problems in your life.
3. Depressions that are caused by an imbalance of chemicals in your brain.

1. Depressions caused by health problems.

One out of every five people who is depressed has a health problem. The way to treat this depression is to treat the health problem.

Here are some health problems which can cause depression:

1. Sickness can make you depressed.

You may be depressed because you are sick, or because you have been sick recently. Infections such as the flu, bronchitis, and hepatitis can make you depressed. Sometimes you will feel depressed for quite a while after your sickness has gone.

2. Drugs can make you depressed.

There are several drugs which can make you depressed. Tell your doctor about all the drugs and medicine you are taking. Some of them may be making you depressed.

Here are some common drugs which can make you feel depressed:

• **Tranquillizers are drugs which can make you depressed.**
Many women take tranquillizers, such as Valium, Ativan, and Librium. They take them to help their "nerves", and to help them sleep. Although tranquillizers are sometimes useful for a short time, many people take them for much too long. Then they cause many side effects. They make people feel drowsy, and tired, and unable to think straight.

Tranquillizers cause even more problems for depressed people. This is because tranquillizers are **depressants**. They make people feel more down and depressed.

If you are depressed, don't take tranquillizers. They will not make you feel better. In fact, they will likely make you feel worse. If you are taking tranquillizers, you will have a harder time solving your problems. Tranquillizers are no help if you are depressed.

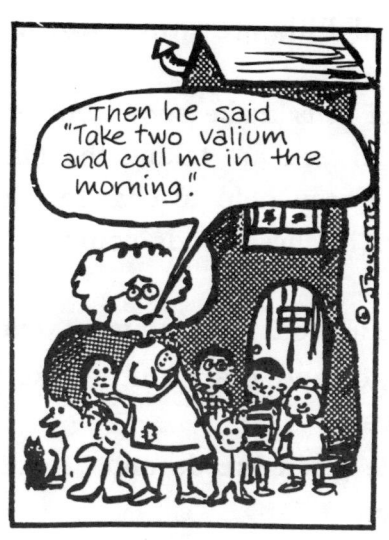

© J. Doucette, 1987

- Alcohol is a drug which can make you depressed.
  Alcohol is also a depressant. You may like to
  drink when you feel down, but this is a mistake.
  Alcohol can make you depressed. And, if you are
  already depressed, it will make you feel worse.
  Don't drink if you are depressed.

If you take tranquillizers and drink alcohol at the
same time, you will certainly feel more depressed.
They both affect your brain in the same way.
Together they make you feel very drowsy. Too
much of them together can even kill you.

- **Birth Control Pills are drugs which can make you depressed.**
  Birth control pills make some women feel depressed. If you are taking the Pill and you are depressed, it may help to change what you eat. Eating more of these foods could help you feel better:
  - more protein foods (hamburger, liver, pork, eggs)
  - more oranges and grapefruit (Take your Pill with orange juice.)
  - more whole grain breads and cereals
  - more peanuts
  - more dark green vegetables (broccoli, spinach)

  If eating these foods doesn't help, you may need a different Pill, or a different kind of birth control.

3. Your hormones can make you depressed.
You may be depressed because your hormones are out of balance. Hormones are chemicals which control parts of your body. For example, sex hormones control your sex organs, and thyroid hormones control how quickly you use up your food. If your body is producing the wrong amount of hormones, you may feel sick. You may also feel depressed.

- You may feel depressed because of a thyroid problem. This can usually be easily treated with thyroid medication.

- You may feel depressed because your female hormone levels are changing. This happens each month before your period starts. During this time, many women feel depressed. Some women feel much worse than others. This kind of depression usually ends when your period starts. This is part of PMS, or Premenstrual Syndrome. (If you want to know more about PMS, please read p. 34, in Chapter 1, Eating Well.)
- You may feel depressed during menopause, when your hormone levels are changing. You may feel up one day and down the next. Or you may feel depressed for longer periods of time. This depression may partly be due to changing hormones. It can also be because your problems as a middle-aged woman aren't taken very seriously. (If you are interested, please read p. 382, Chapter 13, Menopause.)
- You may feel depressed after childbirth. This is called a postpartum depression, or the "baby-blues". This depression may be partly due to changing hormones. It may also be because you are having a hard time coping with the work of a new baby.

You likely will not need drugs if you are depressed because of changing female hormones. You may feel better once you know what is going on.

You may also find it very helpful to talk with other women with the same problem. This is what self-help support groups are for. There are menopause support groups, postpartum groups, thyroid support groups and many others. In these groups you can get support and advice. These groups also give you a chance to spend time with other people who understand your problem.

2. Depressions caused by problems in your life.

You may be depressed because of a problem in your life. If you are seeing a psychiatrist or a therapist, they may call this a "situational depression" or a "reactive depression".

Women face many problems which can make them depressed. Anyone can become depressed if they don't have what they need, and they don't have the power to get it. In our society, many women are in this situation. They don't have what they need, and they don't have the power to get it. This may be why so many women become depressed, especially young, single mothers. This may be why people who are poor and unemployed become depressed. This may be why old people become depressed. This may be why anyone who is being treated unfairly may feel depressed.

Here is a short list of the kinds of problems which can make you depressed. You may have some of these problems or you may have different problems in your life.

- a death of a relative or friend
- a move to a new town
- a new baby
- too much stress
- the loss of a job
- no job except the unpaid job of raising children
- an unhappy marriage
- a violent marriage
- sexual assault or incest
- not enough respect
- not enough money
- not enough friends
- poor housing

If you are depressed because of a problem, a therapist might be very helpful. A therapist might help you solve your problem. A therapist might also be able to help you feel much better. Then you would have more energy to start changing things. Then you would be able to start taking more control of your life.

Some problems can be solved more easily than others. For example, you may be lonely and depressed because you have moved to a new town. If you had support, and if you made some new friends, you would likely feel better.

Or, you may be depressed because you have a violent partner. Battered women often feel depressed, and this certainly makes sense. If you are being battered, you don't need to learn to live with your situation, and you don't need drugs. Your life has to change. Either your partner has to stop hurting you, or you have to leave. After he has stopped hurting you, or you have left, you will start feeling better. When you feel that you can control your own life again, your depression will begin to lift.

It may help to talk with someone before you decide what is best to do. You could call the nearest women's shelter and talk on the phone. If the shelter is far away, there may be a toll-free number you could call. In Ontario you can call the Wife Assault Helpline. It is listed under "W" in the white pages. Crisis centres and the police usually have the number for women's shelters.

We can solve some of our problems by ourselves. However, some of women's problems need to be worked on with others. Many of the problems women face are caused by social problems, such as low incomes and poor housing. These are things which are very hard to solve on our own. These problems need many people working on them together.

Many women in Canada are working on these problems. They are working together to get the things that women need, such as:

- good jobs, and good job-training
- good housing
- good medical care when we are sick, and good information about how to stay well
- an end to violent crimes against women and children
- more day care centres
- more public buildings which are accessible to disabled people
- enough money to provide for our children
- better services for old people
- better services for immigrants
- clean air and water
- world peace

If you started working with other people on these problems, you might make your life better. You might also start to feel better - all at the same time!

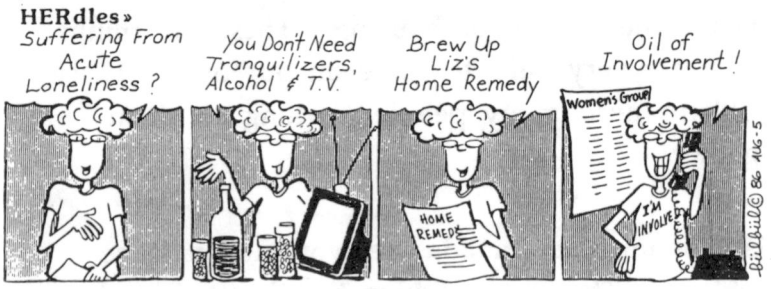

© Bulbul, 1986

3. Depressions caused by an imbalance: biological depressions.

Sometimes people get depressed even when they are healthy, and even when everything is going well in their lives. Doctors think that this kind of depression is caused by an imbalance of chemicals in the brain. They call these depressions "biological depressions".

Doctors treat biological depressions with drugs called anti-depressants. Anti-depressants work well for some people with this kind of depression. They help to balance the chemicals in their brain.

However, anti-depressants are only useful for biological depressions. They are useless for depressions which are caused by health problems or problems in your life. However, many doctors prescribe them before they are sure if the person has a biological depression. Doctors give them to many people who do not have biological depressions.

Anti-depressants are strong drugs, and they can produce unpleasant side effects. When people who don't need anti-depressants take them, they often end up feeling worse. They have to put up with the side effects, without getting any help for their depression. Then it is hard to tell if they are depressed because of their situation, or because of the drugs.

There are several reasons why anti-depressants are prescribed too often.
- A biological depression is not easy to diagnose. If you have a biological depression you will not feel like your "old self". Like any depressed person, you may have changes in your appetite and in how much you sleep. You may notice changes in your energy, and in how well you can think. You may have changes in your moods, and in your interest in sex. You may feel worthless and you may think about suicide. These feelings can last for a very long time.

Many people with situational depressions have the very same symptoms. Your symptoms alone won't tell you if you need an anti-depressant.

- **There is no test to prove if you need an anti-depressant.**
  The only way a doctor can decide if you might need an anti-depressant is by understanding your depression as well as possible. This takes time to do. This would take several visits with your doctor over several weeks. Some doctors don't take enough time to understand your depression, and they prescribe too quickly.
- **Many doctors are not trained in therapy.**
  They often don't know what else to do for someone who is depressed except give them pills.
- **Many patients and many doctors are used to thinking of pills as good answers to health problems.**

Before you decide to take an anti-depressant talk with your doctor several times. At these visits tell your doctor as much as you can about how you feel. Your doctor should make sure that no other problem is making you depressed. Then, if no other problem in your life can be blamed, you and your doctor may decide that you have a biological depression. Then you may want to take an anti-depressant to help you.

Using anti-depressants safely:

There are three common kinds of anti-depressants:
- tricyclics, such as imipramine and amitriptyline
- MAO inhibitors
- lithium.

There are several things you should know about these pills:

1. Anti-depressants are strong drugs.
Anti-depressants can produce many serious side-effects. Side effects are extra ways that a drug affects you. Some of the side effects of anti-depressants are a dry mouth, constipation, nausea, headaches, sleeping problems, dizziness, and tiredness. Pregnant women should never take anti-depressants.

Your doctor must take the time to explain the side effects you might have. Your doctor should tell you how long they will last, and what you can do about them.

2. Anti-depressants work slowly.
You will likely have to take anti-depressants for several weeks before you feel any better. If they are working, you should feel good after 4 to 6 weeks. Be sure to see your doctor regularly during this time. Once they have started to work, you shouldn't feel drugged or high. You should feel more like your old self.

If you don't feel any better after 6 weeks, then they aren't working. You likely need to stop taking them and to try a different treatment.

3. Anti-depressants must be taken regularly.
Follow the instructions on the label very carefully and take them regularly.
Never take anti-depressants now and again when you are feeling a little down.

4. It is easy to over-dose on anti-depressants.
An over-dose often causes death.

5. Don't drink alcohol if you are taking anti-depressants.
Anti-depressants plus alcohol can cause serious problems. You must also avoid certain foods and certain other drugs while you are taking some anti-depressants.

6. Go off them gradually, if you decide to stop taking anti-depressants.
If you stop taking anti-depressants suddenly, you might feel quite sick. Talk with your doctor about how to stop taking them, and follow the directions carefully.

Before you decide to take an anti-depressant think carefully.

- Make sure that no other problem in your life is making you depressed.
- If you decide to take them, learn about the side-effects.
- While you are taking them, see your doctor regularly.
- If you wish, you may also want to go for therapy while you are taking the anti-depressants.

Anti-depressants are useful when they help people feel better. Anti-depressants are a problem when they are given to people who don't need them. When depressed people only get a strong drug which they don't need, they miss out. They miss out on the therapy or the friendship and support which they really need.

Remember: being depressed does not mean that you are crazy. Anyone can be depressed. Being depressed just means that something is wrong. If you get help, you can feel good again. If you do not get the help you need, you may feel even worse. Get the help you need so you can start enjoying your life again. Getting help is a sign of strength, not of weakness. Even if you have to push yourself to go for help, do it!! You may not believe it now, but **you need some help, and you deserve it**.

Getting help for your depression.

"Who should I talk to?"

You could talk with a therapist, a social worker, or a counsellor. You could also talk with a member of the clergy, a psychologist, or a psychiatrist. You could also join a self-help group.

If you want to find a good therapist, the best way is to ask around.

- Ask someone who has been depressed. Ask them who they talked to.
- Ask your doctor or your public health nurse to recommend someone.
- Ask the local Canadian Mental Health Association.
- Ask a Women's Referral Centre.
- Ask a Family Counselling Service. Family Counselling Services have counsellors who will see you by yourself or with members of your family. Their fees are very low or free for people with low incomes.

Finding the right therapist for you is a very personal thing. The therapist who is best for you may not be best for someone else.

Here are some things to look for in a good therapist:

1. Someone who will help you cope on your own.
You need to find someone who will help you to cope better on your own. You don't want a therapist who solves your problems for you. You want one who teaches you to solve your problems. And, you want a therapist who supports you while you change parts of your life. After a while, you shouldn't need your therapist any more.

2. Someone who won't blame you.
You need to find someone who won't judge you or blame you for whatever has happened.

3. Someone who doesn't just give out drugs.
You need to find someone who doesn't just give you prescriptions for drugs. Some drugs can be useful for some people, but often they are not enough by themselves.

4. Someone who knows how to deal with stress.
You need to find someone who will teach you better ways to cope with daily stress.

5. **Someone who you can afford.**

You need someone you can afford. Psychiatrists and some psychologists are covered by provincial medical plans. Other therapists are not covered, and you will have to pay them yourself. Some therapists have a "sliding scale". This means that they charge according to how much people can afford.

6. **Someone who knows about problems like yours.**

You need to find someone who has had experience dealing with problems like yours. You may want to ask them about how long they have been a therapist, and how many clients they have had. You may also want to ask the therapist about their training before you start going to them.

7. **Someone you are comfortable with.**

You may want the person to be a woman, or you may want a man, or you may not care either way. Be sure you are comfortable with the person you chose. Be sure that you feel that you can trust this person.

Although it doesn't happen often, once in a while a therapist will tell his client that she should have sex with him. The therapist says that sex will help solve her problems. This is wrong. A therapist who says this is lying to you, and you should report him. It is a good idea to get a lawyer to help you do this. Ask Legal Aid for help.

8. **Someone who is concerned about women.**

You may want to find someone who is aware of the special problems women have in our society. Your depression may be connected to how you have been treated as a woman.

If you are not happy with what is going on with your therapist, tell her or him. You may be able to work out your problem. Or, you may need to find a different therapist. Just like with doctors, you have the right to ask questions, and the right to get answers which you can understand.

At the therapist's.

"What's going to happen?"

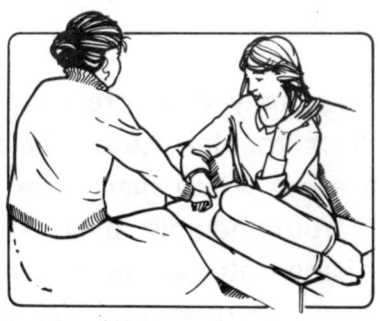

You and your therapist need to figure out why you are depressed. To do this, your therapist will have to ask you lots of questions. The therapist needs to know what your life has been like so you both can figure out where your problems started.

Your therapist will likely ask about the important people in your life, such as your family and your friends. She or he may want to know about your health, and your work, and your hobbies.

At first, you might feel upset when you talk about your problems. After a few times, it will likely get much easier. You may find that when you talk about upsetting things, you can learn new ways to get over them.

Therapists and counsellors are very helpful for depressions which are caused by problems in your life. A good therapist will help you to understand your situation. He or she may also help you solve your problem. After talking with your therapist, you may learn to see things in a different light. You may also learn some new ways to behave.

For example, you may be depressed since your divorce. Perhaps you feel guilty for not making your marriage work. You may think that you were a "bad wife". Your therapist may show you that it is wrong to blame only one person when a marriage falls apart. Your therapist might also show you that you need to change some of your ideas about what a "bad wife" is. Your therapist may show you that feeling guilty keeps you from getting on with the rest of your life.

Most people who are depressed think that they are not worthwhile people. Your therapist may call this having "low self-esteem". Your therapist will likely try to make you see how important you are. When you start to feel more worthwhile, then things won't get you down so much. You will have more energy to deal with your problems. You will begin to have more control over your life.

In order to improve your self-esteem, you usually need to change some of your **ideas**, and you need to change some of the ways you **act**. Your therapist will help you look at your ideas about yourself. You will see which ideas are helpful to you and which are not. Your therapist should also support you while you learn new ways to think. Your therapist should also support you if you need to learn new ways to behave. These new ways may help you to work on the problems in your life. Besides a therapist, you may also want to go to a support group for extra help.

Remember: even if you want them, these changes may be hard and slow and painful. If you are making big changes in how you live your life, it is never quick or easy. But it is worth it.

These are some new things you may have to learn:
- New ways to take care of yourself.
- New ways to know what you need, and how to get it for yourself.
- New ways to see the good things about yourself.
- New ways to see the good things you have done over the years. In other words, you will learn how to appreciate yourself.
- New ways to notice how you put yourself down, and how to stop doing this.
- New ways to handle stress in your life. (If you want more information on dealing with stress, please read Chapter 2, <u>Dealing With Your "Nerves"</u>.)

You may also have to learn:
- New ways to act with the people you have trouble with.
- New ways to understand things that have happened to you so that you can prevent them from happening again.
- New ways to understand how you have been treated as a woman, and how this has affected you.

In other words, you will be learning new ways to take control of your life.

Depression is serious. Don't try and cope with it alone. When you are depressed you can get help, and you can get better. There are good people out there who can give you the help that you need and deserve.

Being Active

4

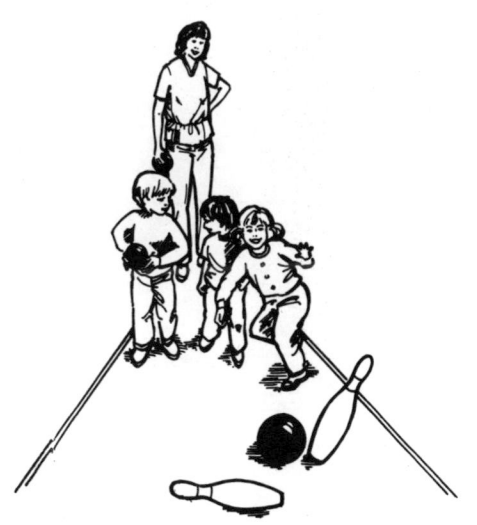

BEING ACTIVE

Being active is one of the cheapest and best things you can do for your health.

Our bodies are meant to move. Remember how much children move around, just because they like to. As adults, most of us don't use our bodies very much. We use cars and buses instead of walking. We watch sports instead of playing them. We have learned to be inactive, and we need to learn to be active again.

Fitness is not just for athletes. Fitness is for all of us. The basic idea about fitness is **being active.** That's all there is to it. You can walk, bicycle, swim or dance. You can play a sport, or dig in the garden, or scrub the floor. As long as you don't overdo it, being active can help you feel better.

If you keep active, then you will have lots of energy. If you don't, then you may get tired easily. So, if you are tired a lot of the time, this could be a sign that you are not active enough. You likely don't need more rest. You likely need to be more active. Strange as this may seem, being active can give you **more energy.**

"What can being active really do for me?"

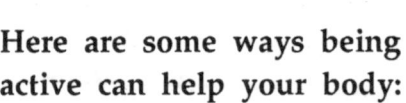

Being active can make you feel good. Being active can make your body and your mind work better.

Here are some ways being active can help your body:

1) Being active gives you energy, so you can work well without getting tired.

2) Being active is a good way to help control high blood pressure. It also helps to prevent hardening of the arteries, which can lead to high blood pressure and heart disease.

3) Being active keeps your heart strong. This helps prevent heart disease.

4) Being active makes your muscles stronger. Lower back pain, for example, can be caused by weak muscles.

5) Being active makes your joints more flexible, so you can move more easily.

6) Being active helps make your bones stronger and thicker. This is very important as you grow older.

7) Being active helps you to be thin. It helps you use up extra fat. If you exercise regularly, you will burn fat both while you are exercising and while you are resting.

Here are some ways being active can help your mind work better:

1) An active person can handle stress better. Too much stress can be harmful. It can lead to headaches and ulcers. It can make you feel very tired. Exercise helps you get rid of the harmful effects of stress, because it acts like a natural, safe tranquillizer. It gives your body a chance to relax safely. It helps you take your mind off your problems for a while. It also calms you down so you can get a good sleep. Next time you are feeling uptight, try something active. Go for a walk, or dig in the garden, or wash the floor. Don't have a pill or a drink. Then see how you feel. Being active may work for you.

2) Being active can help you feel better when you are depressed.

3) Being active can make your body stronger. When your body is stronger, you may feel stronger and more able to deal with your problems.

4) Being active is a way to get time by yourself.

5) Being active can make you feel better and look better. You will have more energy for your work, for yourself and for your children.

Think about the difference being active could make for you!

"I really want to be more active but...."
Does this sound familiar??

Famous excuses and how to get around them:

"I'm embarrassed because I'm too fat (or too thin or too awkward or....)"
Everyone feels some of this at first. It will go away. If you are embarrassed, you could start exercising at home alone.

"It takes too much time."
The best way is to be active for 15 minutes, 3 times a week. Smaller amounts of exercise will also make you feel better. At first, you may have to make time to exercise. After a while, it will become a habit.

"I'm too tired."
You may be tired because you need to be more active. Believe it or not, exercising will give you energy. If you start exercising, you'll be less tired in a few weeks, or even a few days.

"My appetite will increase, and I'll eat more and get fat!"

Being active helps control your appetite. Instead of gaining, you'll likely start losing.

"It'll hurt too much."

Exercise shouldn't hurt. There is a big difference between feeling the exercise and feeling pain. If you have a pain, check that you are doing the exercise properly. If the pain lasts, check with your doctor.

Be sure that you are wearing good running shoes which support your feet well. If you stretch before you exercise you will prevent many injuries, and you won't be sore afterwards. Be sure to do some stretching before and after very active exercise, such as skating or jogging. Stretch the muscles in your upper and lower legs.

Most people start off doing too much the first day. Then they are so sore the next day that they never want to move again. This kind of pain comes from over-doing it. Go easy at first. Then do a little more every day.

"I can't get around to it."

Set a regular time just for exercise and stick to it. Think how good you will feel afterwards.

"I don't have the right clothes. I can't afford tights or a jogging suit."
You don't have to have special clothes or special equipment to be active. All you need are comfortable clothes and good light shoes which support your feet.

"It's a good idea, but there are more important things I should be doing for my family."
Being active regularly is not a selfish thing to do. It will help you stay healthy and make you feel good. Your family needs you to be healthy. And if you feel good, then you can help others feel good too.

Getting Started.

"Should I check with my doctor before I begin?"
1) Check with your doctor if you are over 40 and have not exercised regularly.

2) Check with your doctor if you have any of these health problems:
- high blood pressure
- heart or chest pains
- faintness or dizziness
- frequent headaches
- back or knee problems
- arthritis
- more than 50 pounds of extra weight

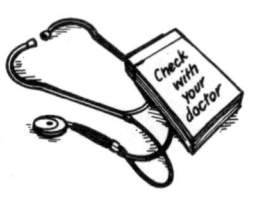

3) Check with your doctor if you are taking any medication. Ask your doctor if any exercises are not safe while you are taking this drug. Your doctor should also tell you what warning signs to watch for while you are exercising.

If you have a health problem, you need to know which sports or exercises are safe for you. You could talk about this with your doctor or with a person who teaches fitness. There are fitness instructors who work for most YWCAs, community colleges, community centres, and boards of education.

To help you get started, ask yourself these questions:
- Why do I want to be more active?
- What do I want to do?
- When do I want to do it?

1) *"Why do I want to be more active?"*
Perhaps you want to lose weight, or you want to have more energy. Perhaps you want to do something about your bad nerves.

Remember why you want to be more active. This will give you a reason to keep at it, even when you don't feel like it.

2) "What do I want to do?"

Here are some questions to help you figure out what you want to do:

- What sports or activities have you enjoyed doing in the past?
- Which sports have always looked like fun?
- Which activities could easily fit into your life?
- What kind of person are you? Do you like to be alone, or would you rather do things with other people?

Here are some activities and sports you could do, either on your own or with others:

Activities to do on your own:

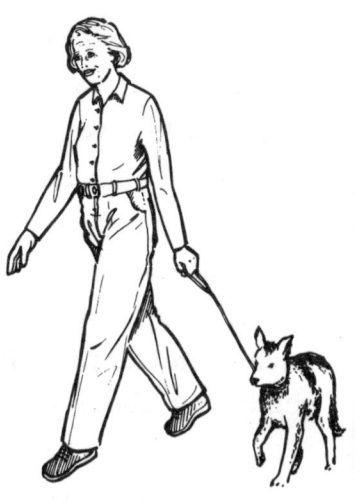

- walk (Walking is easy, safe, handy and cheap.)
- swim
- bicycle
- skate
- jog (Only jog if you have good shoes.)
- dance by yourself at home
- exercise with TV fitness shows

Activities to do with others:

- play with your children: play tag, or baseball, or frisbee
- swim
- ice-skate or roller-skate
- bowl
- play tennis or badminton
- get an exercise record or video, and do it together with your friends
- join a baseball team

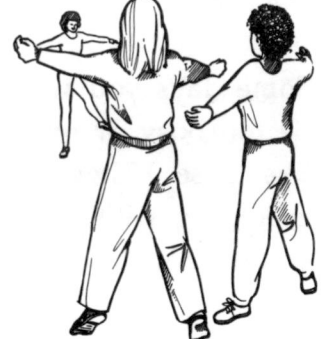

Activities with a class or group:

- a fitness class. Be careful: exercises can cause injuries if they are not done correctly. Be sure your instructor is well trained. You could start with a "low-impact" or "no-impact" class. These exercises are easier on the body.

- a dancersize class
- a dancing class - jazz dancing, square dancing, folk dancing, or even ballet dancing. There are classes given by YWCAs, community centres, and school boards. Many of them have free childcare. Some of them have special rates for people with lower incomes.

3) *"When do I want to do it?"*
After you know why you want to exercise and what you want to do, then you need to decide when to do it.

If you exercise alone, try to make it a habit. Try to set aside the same time each day or each week. Don't change it unless it is a real emergency This way you, your family and friends will take your exercise time seriously.

Some days you won't feel like exercising. You may be too busy or too tired. A friend is useful at times like these. They may be able to "talk you into" exercising with them. Usually, once you get started, you'll be glad you did.

If you don't have time to play a sport or to join a fitness class, you can still get some exercise. If you can't do a lot; do a little. **Do more of what you already do.**

Some every-day things you could do:

- Do some more walking. Get off the bus a few blocks before your stop, and walk the rest of the way. Walk with your friend, or your children, or your dog. Take a break. Go for a walk alone.
- If you're going less than 10 blocks, walk. Save the bus or taxi money and buy yourself a treat.
- Don't use the elevator if you are only going up a few floors. Try running up the stairs sometimes.
- Try walking faster than usual. Try this while you are pushing the baby carriage.
- Play sports with your children.
- Do exercise while watching TV.
- Try doing your gardening or raking a little more quickly than usual. Sweep or vacuum faster.
- Stretch as often as you can. Stretching your muscles is very good for them. See if you can put something on the top shelf without using a chair. Stretch when you pick up after your children. Stretch to hang up the clothes. Stretch your arms and legs in the morning before you get up; it will help you wake up. Stretch in bed at night; it will help you relax.

You'll be able to think of many more ways to get moving. Try them and you will feel less dragged out at the end of the day.

"Is there anything else I need to know?"
Here are a few things to remember so that you don't hurt yourself:

Rules for exercising safely:

- Go easy at first!

Start off slowly, especially if you are not in good shape. If you do too much, too soon, you can hurt yourself. Then you may feel worse, instead of better. Then you may quit too soon. Don't be afraid to work at your own pace. Listen to your body. If it hurts, go slower.

- Build up gradually.

If you want to run, don't run five miles on the first day. Go a short distance at first. Then, little by little, go further. Your body can be trained to be quite strong, but it will take some time. Go slowly.

- Give yourself the "talk test".

When you exercise your heart will beat faster, and your breathing will be quicker. But, if you can still talk while you are exercising, you are not overdoing it. If you can't talk, slow down!

- Always warm up beforehand.

Warm up for about 5 minutes by doing a lot of stretching. This warms up your muscles so they won't be easily hurt.

- Always cool down after exercising.
Slowly walk and stretch until your heart rate is normal again.   This should take about 5 minutes.
You'll feel much better afterwards if you do.
- If you are not sure about what to do, get some advice.   Talk it over with a trained fitness instructor, or your public health nurse, or your doctor.

Smoking and exercise.

If you are a smoker, there are a few things you should know.

1) Smokers cannot do as much exercise as nonsmokers.   This is because smoking affects your lungs.   Smoking makes your lungs less able to send oxygen to your blood.   It also makes your blood less able to carry oxygen.   Smoking is also hard on your heart.

If you smoke, exercise is very important.   Exercise can slow down some of the damage done by smoking.   But exercise alone cannot make up for all the harm done by cigarettes.

2) If you are trying to quit smoking, keep active. Keeping active is a great way to pass the time while you are quitting.

3) If you quit smoking, your body will be healthier. You won't be able to see how much healthier your lungs are. However, you will feel better, and you will have more energy.

4) If you are a smoker and if you are over 35, birth control pills can be dangerous for you. If you take the Pill, you have a greater chance of serious heart disease or stroke. Exercise cannot make up for this danger. Either the Pill or the smoking - or both - have to go. (If you want more information about birth control pills and smoking, please read p. 289, Chapter 9, <u>Birth Control</u>.)

Next time you are tired and you want coffee and a cigarette, try something different. Do some stretching. Start moving and get your heart beating more quickly. Before long, you'll feel less tired and more alert.

If you want to quit smoking, you could get in touch with The Canadian Cancer Society, or The Lung Association, or The Heart and Stroke Association. Some community colleges also have courses to help people quit smoking.

How being active helps during pregnancy.

There are many good reasons for pregnant women to be active. Exercise can improve the baby's health and the mother's health.

This is how your exercise can improve your baby's health:

A growing baby needs a good supply of food and oxygen, and it needs to have its wastes removed. The baby depends on your body to do these things. All the baby's food and oxygen is brought by your blood, and all its wastes are removed by your blood. This is why good blood flow to the baby is so important.

When you are active, your heart pumps faster. This makes your blood move better. The better your blood travels around your body, the better it can carry food and oxygen to your baby. When you are active, your baby will get more of what it needs to be healthy.

Safe exercise helps your baby. It doesn't hurt it. So, don't worry. You will not be using up oxygen your baby needs. And you will not cause a miscarriage. Instead, you will be helping your baby get what it needs.

This is how your exercise improves your health:

- Exercise helps you handle labour and delivery better. Childbirth is hard work. If you exercise, your muscles and your heart and lungs will be used to doing hard work. Regular walking is one of the best ways to prepare for labour.

- Exercise helps you recover more quickly after your baby is born. It also helps you get back into shape more easily.

- Exercise helps prevent you from gaining too much weight. (A pregnant woman should gain 25 to 35 pounds.)

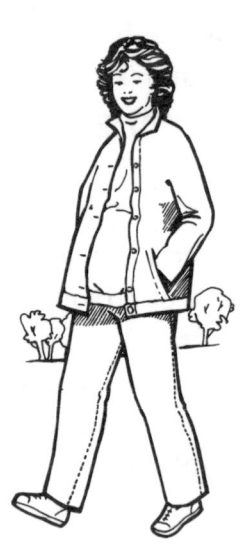

- Exercise makes your muscles stronger. This makes it easier to carry the weight of the baby.

- Exercise helps prevent varicose veins and constipation.

- Exercise helps you relax and sleep better. It also gives you more energy so you will feel less tired.

"I'm pregnant and I'm not sure what exercise to do."

1) Start by getting some advice from your doctor or public health nurse. If you are going to a prenatal class, ask your instructor. You need to know which exercises are safe to do and which aren't. Some exercises put too much strain on your back and stomach muscles.

2) **If it hurts, don't do it.** Listen to your body.

3) If you want to join a fitness program, join a prenatal fitness class.

4) If you want to exercise on your own, do a little exercise several times a day. You don't need to do anything fancy. Go for good, long walks. A half-hour walk, three or four times a week, will help you feel better.

Rest is good when you are pregnant, and so is exercise. Don't spend too much time with your "feet up". Get active!

How being active helps during menstruation.

Many of us were told long ago not to do any exercise during our periods. Now we know that this is not good advice. For some women, exercise helps them get rid of menstrual cramps. Others find that their breasts and stomach swell up less before their periods if they exercise. Others say it helps them to get rid of the "blues" before their periods.

Next time you have your period try some gentle stretching followed by a long walk. You may feel much better if you do.

How being active helps during menopause.

Exercise is useful for women at all ages. Women over 35 have another good reason to be more active. During and after menopause, our bones start to lose some of their calcium. This makes them thinner and more breakable. This is called "osteoporosis".

Exercise is one of the best ways to prevent thinning of the bones. Exercise makes our bones stronger. (There is much more information on osteoporosis on p. 378, in Chapter 13, <u>Menopause</u>.)

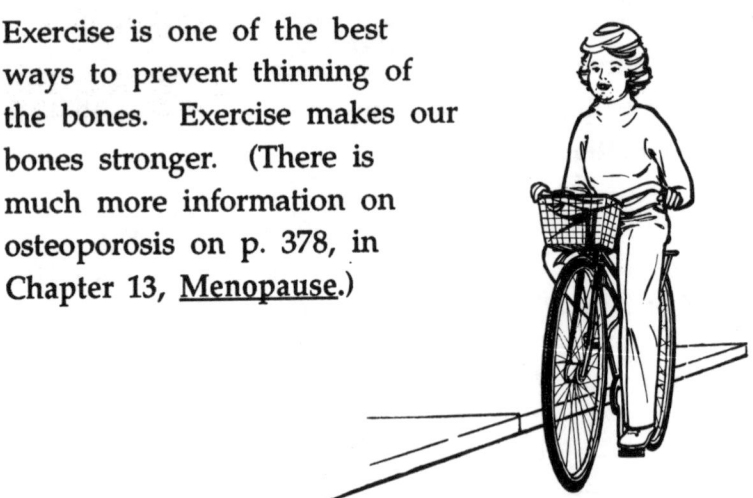

Being active is one of the best things you can do for your health.

Controlling
Your Weight

5

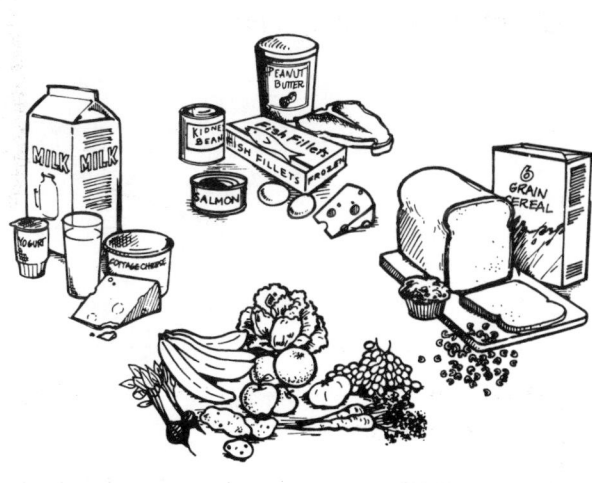

CONTROLLING YOUR WEIGHT

Many people in North America think that women must be beautiful to be lovable. And in North America, most people think that to be beautiful, you must be thin.

As a result, many of us spend a huge amount of our time and money trying to be thin. Women spend millions of dollars on diets, drinks, gadgets, operations, and diet pills. Besides costing time and money, most of these things are useless. Even worse, many of them are dangerous.

Dieting is a good example of something harmful which many women do. Year after year, thousands and thousands of women eat much less food than their bodies need. Year after year, they starve themselves. They end up feeling sick, tired, and depressed. And, if their diets don't work, they end up hating themselves for being fat.

How much fat is too much fat?

The big question is: "How much fat is too much fat?" If we compare ourselves to the women on TV, we may think that any extra fat is awful. This is a mistake. Extra fat is only a problem when it hurts your health.

There is a lot of pressure on us to be thin, and we need to be aware it. We need to think carefully about how important it really is to be thin. We need to think carefully about who benefits most from our trying to be thin. If you are worried about your weight, think about why you want to lose weight. You need to be sure that you have a good reason to lose weight.

Good reasons to lose weight.

There are only two good reasons to lose weight: to improve your health, and to feel better.

1. To improve your health.
The best reason to lose weight is to improve your health. You don't have to be thin to be healthy. However, too much extra fat can cause problems.

Over the years, doctors have changed their opinions about how much fat is too much. Many doctors now think that you can safely have 30 to 40 pounds of extra fat. If you have more than 40 extra pounds, you will have a higher risk of getting these diseases:

- diabetes
- heart disease
- varicose veins
- cancer in your breast, bowel or uterus
- joint problems
- high blood pressure
- gall bladder problems

If you are worried about how much you weigh, talk with your doctor or your public health nurse. Find out if your weight is dangerous to your health.

Your doctor or nurse may use the B.M.I. (Body Mass Index) to figure out if you are overweight. This is an easy way to know if you are a healthy weight for your height.

Some doctors are like many people in our society; they hate fatness, especially in women. These doctors might pressure you to lose weight, even if you are only a few pounds overweight. If your doctor wants you to lose weight, find out why. Find out if your extra weight is a real risk to your health.

2. To Feel Better.
The other good reason to lose weight is to feel better. If you weighed less, you might feel better. You might have much more energy, and you might find it easier to move around.

Losing weight to improve your health or to feel better are good reasons to lose weight.

Bad reasons to lose weight.

1. So you will be happy.

Being thin won't solve all your problems. Being thin won't guarantee that you will be happy for the rest of your life. Being thin won't guarantee that you'll find a perfect partner, or a perfect job. Many fat people are beautiful and happy, and many thin people are not.

2. So someone will love you.

Don't try to lose weight to please someone else. Often a partner or a friend or a relative will tell you that you should lose weight. Sometimes they say this because they want you to look a certain way. They think that if you look a certain way, then they will be happy.

Before you decide to lose weight, ask yourself why you want to. If you think losing weight will make someone love you more, think again. If you think losing weight will make someone treat you better, or even stay with you, think again. Your value as a person comes from who you are, not from how you look.

Why some of us are over-weight.

1. We don't get enough exercise.

Most people who are fat are not active enough. If you don't move around enough, you won't use up all the energy in your food. The extra energy is stored as fat.

Many fat people do not eat more than thin people do. They just move a lot less than thinner people do.

2. We eat more high-calorie foods than we can use up.

Calories measure the amount of energy in your food. If a food has a lot of calories, then it contains a lot of energy. If you eat more calories than you use up, then your body will store the extra calories as fat. This is why too much high-calorie food can make you fat.

People use up their food at different speeds. Some people use up food quickly, and some don't. Some people easily store the extra as fat, and some don't.

People who eat lots without ever gaining weight use up their food quickly. They also do not store fat very well. People who gain weight easily, even on a diet, use up their food slowly. They also store fat well.

Here are a few reasons why some people use up their food more slowly than others:

- People who are not very active use up their food more slowly.
- People who are older use up their food more slowly.
- People who have always been fat may have bodies which use up food slowly.
- People who have been on many low-calorie diets often use up their food slowly.

3. **Dieting.**
Strange as it sounds, a lot of dieting can make you fat. Here is what happens.

If there were a famine and you were starving, your body would change the way it used its food. It would do this to make up for the lack of food. First, your body would begin to use up your food more slowly. Then it would also begin to store fat for the future. This is your body's way of trying to keep you from losing so much weight that you would die.

When you go on a low-calorie diet, your body acts as if you were starving. First your body starts to use up your food more slowly. Then it starts to use up your body fat more slowly. It also tries to store fat for the future. The less you eat, the less food and fat your body uses up. The less you eat, the more fat it tries to store. This is why low-calorie diets often don't work. This is why you can be on a diet and still not lose very much weight.

When you go off your diet, your body may return to normal. You may start to use up your food more quickly again. However, you may have another problem. Your body may continue as if you were still on a diet - as if you were still starving. It will continue to use up your food slowly. Then you will quickly gain back the weight you lost. And, you may go on gaining until you end up heavier than before you began dieting.

If you have been on many diets, your body may be good at storing fat and using food slowly. Your body may have learned how to keep your weight steady. If this has happened to you, exercise can be very helpful. Exercise helps your body to start using up your food more quickly.

4. Some other reasons why some of us are fat.

- Some women like being large and powerful.
  They enjoy taking up more space than women are "supposed" to.
- Some women have decided to rebel against the way we are "supposed" to look. They don't want to spend a lot of time trying to look a certain way to please others.
  They like themselves the way they are.
- Some people have medical problems which make them gain weight.

Ask your doctor if your weight is harmful to your health. If it is, then you should likely lose some weight. If it is not, then you decide for yourself whether or not you want to lose weight.

Ways to lose weight that are safe.

If you want to lose weight safely:
1) Be more active.
2) Eat good food.
3) Change some of your old eating habits.

1) **Be more active and lose weight safely**.

One of the very best ways to lose weight safely is to become more active.

"How can exercise help me lose weight?"

- Exercise does a wonderful thing. It makes your body use up your food more quickly.

- Exercise helps you to control your appetite so you will only want the amount of food you really need. Exercise will **not** make you eat more than ever.

- Exercise helps by making your body need more energy. Your body can get this energy from your extra fat.

- Exercise helps you get rid of stress. If you don't feel as uptight, then you might not eat to make yourself feel better. Exercise is a great treatment for "the blues".

- Exercise helps you to be able to eat high-calorie treats now and again. If you are active your body can use up the extra calories more easily.

- Exercise helps tone up your muscles so you will look firmer.

- Exercise helps you to feel better and to have more energy.
  Here's how: Some people did an experiment to find out the effects of exercise. They asked some college students to do two different things. Some days they asked them to go for a quick ten-minute walk. Other days they asked them to eat a candy bar and rest for ten minutes instead.

The students said that they felt much better on the days that they walked. They said they had more energy and they felt less tense. They said that they felt full of energy for two hours after the walk. Remember this when you are tired and want a candy bar. Take a walking break instead.

When you are exercising and eating low-calorie foods, you may expect to lose weight quickly. This may not happen. This is because your muscles may be growing. Muscles weigh more than fat.

If you want to find out if you are thinner, don't weigh yourself. Measure your waist instead. If it is smaller, then you have less fat, even if you do not weigh much less.

"What exercises should I do?"

Exercise doesn't have to be
fancy. If you are very
overweight, one of the best
exercises is a brisk, 20 minute
daily walk. It is cheap and
easy. This is one of the best
ways for a heavy person to
start an exercise program.

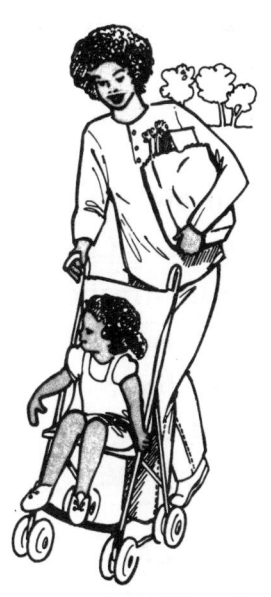

Don't start off with anything
more active, like running, until
you are used to regular brisk
walking. Get some advice
from your doctor or public
health nurse. Find out if your
heart is healthy enough for
more active exercise.

Exercise just means being active. It doesn't mean
that you have to join a special exercise program. It
means walking instead of taking a bus or a taxi. It
means riding a bike or going swimming. Make time
in your life for some exercise and you will feel
better. You may also lose some extra fat.

If you want information about how to be more
active, you could read Chapter 4, Being Active.

2) Eat good food and lose weight safely.

"What should I eat?"

• First of all, make sure you are eating a **balanced diet**. A balanced diet is not a low-calorie diet. Forget about low-calorie diets, and think about balanced diets instead. You need good food to be healthy.

If you are not sure how to eat a balanced diet, please read Chapter 1, <u>Eating Well</u>. If you want more information, talk with your doctor or your public health nurse. You can also get advice from a nutritionist or a dietitian at a hospital.

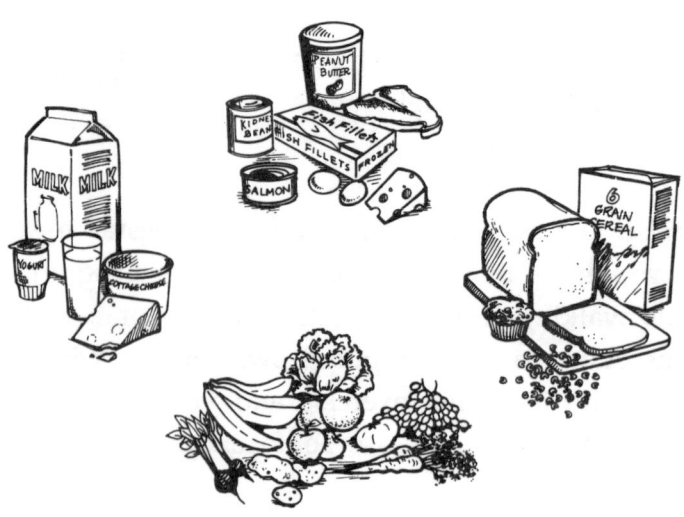

- Eat a good breakfast and a good lunch. These meals give you energy to get through the day. [People who skip breakfast often overeat at other meals. They also often eat high-calorie snacks during the day.]
Unless you are very active in the evening, eat a light supper. If you don't use up the extra calories from supper, they will be stored as fat.

- Eat more foods containing fibre. Fibre is found in whole grains, cereals, fruit and vegetables. Fibre is good because it fills you up without a lot of calories. It also helps prevent constipation.

- Eat fewer foods containing fat. Fat is very high in calories. There is a lot of fat in butter, margarine, ice cream, cream cheese, wieners, cold cuts, deep fried foods and chips. For example: an order of fried chicken and fries, contains as many calories as you may need in a whole day!!

- When you are cooking, use as little fat as you can. Drain off extra fat. Trim off fat from meat. Before cooking chicken pieces, remove the skin. Instead of frying, broil meats. Use a non-stick pan so you don't need to use fat to fry. Cook some foods in a little water, instead of in fat.

- Drink lots of water.

"How can eating good food help me lose weight?"

- If you fill up on good food, you will have no room left for high-calorie snacks.
- If you eat good food, you will have lots of energy to be active. Active people use up body fat more easily.
- If you eat good food, you will feel good. Then you won't often feel depressed, and you won't want high-calorie snacks to cheer yourself up.

3) Change some of your old eating habits and lose weight safely.

Here are some new ways to eat:
- Avoid fast foods such as hamburgers, fish and chips, and donuts. These foods contain lots of fat, which means lots of calories.
- Don't skip breakfast and lunch.
- Don't drink high calorie foods like alcohol and pop with your meals.
- Don't put high-calorie things on your food. If you are trying to lose weight, use very little of these foods: gravy, salad dressings, mayonnaise, butter, sour cream.
  Use these instead: lemon juice, low-calorie dressings, yogurt, spices.

- Keep lots of raw fruit and vegetables handy for when you get hungry.
- Get rid of junk food. Start eating good food all the time.
- Learn some new ways of taking care of yourself besides high-calorie treats. Try having long baths, or visiting with a friend, or listening to music, or going for walks. Find the ways that work for you.
- Don't eat because you are upset, or bored, or angry.
- Don't eat at the movies or when you watch TV.
- Skip dessert.
- Stop eating as soon as you are full. You don't have to clean off your plate.
- Don't eat up everyone else's leftovers so food isn't "wasted".
- Don't go shopping when you are hungry. If you do, you will buy food that you shouldn't eat. Don't buy sweet treats for yourself or your family.
- Get as much support as you can. It isn't easy at first to change old eating habits. If you get support from your family and friends it can make a big difference.

- Above all: Don't starve yourself. Don't go on any more low-calorie diets.

  Dieting can be both dangerous and useless. It is not healthy to have your weight going up and down. Many people feel lousy while they are dieting. Many people feel tired, cranky, and depressed. Others feel dizzy, and have headaches. Many say that they can't think clearly, and that they get sick more often. This is not a good way to live!

  Because they feel so bad, nearly all people quit their diets. And when they do, they soon gain back the weight they lost. Diets are not the answer to controlling your weight.

Don't be discouraged. If you eat good food you will lose weight. You will lose it slowly but surely, and you will feel good.

Ways to lose weight that are not safe.

Because we worry so much about being thin, many of us want a magic, quick way to lose weight. Many women try to lose weight with useless and sometimes dangerous methods. When it comes to losing weight, quick answers just don't work.

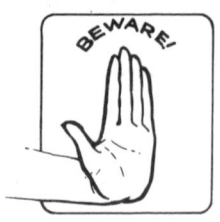

Here is some information about some **dangerous** ways to lose weight:

1) Crash diets and fad diets are dangerous.
Some diets tell you that "you can lose 30 pounds in 3 weeks!" These "crash diets" or "fad diets" are unbalanced diets. They are dangerous because they do not give you the foods you need. They don't give you enough energy, protein, vitamins and minerals. These kinds of diets put a great strain on your body.

No serious damage will happen after a few days of eating an unbalanced diet. But, if you eat an unbalanced diet for weeks and weeks, then your body will start to break down.

For example, if you don't eat enough protein, then your body will start to break itself down to get this protein. You will lose muscle cells from all over your body. Your hair will not look healthy and you will not feel healthy. You will feel tired, dizzy and depressed.

Besides making you feel bad, these diets don't work. No one can stay on them for very long. Most people gain back the weight they have lost soon after they stop the diet.

2) Drugs to lose weight are dangerous.

Diet pills, or "appetite suppressants", speed up your body and take away your appetite. Going without food is dangerous, and so are diet pills.

- Diet pills can cause dangerous high blood pressure.
- Diet pills can make you feel very nervous.
- Diet pills can be addictive.
- Diet pills can cause very unpleasant withdrawal symptoms when you stop taking them.
- Diet pills must only be taken after you have checked with your doctor.
- Diet pills must only be taken for a short time, if they are taken at all.

Some diet pills contain only a large dose of caffeine. They can make you feel very nervous and on edge.

Using pills will not help you understand why you are fat. They will also not help you stay thin. They are dangerous. Avoid them.

Some women use diuretics ("water pills"). They think these pills will help them lose weight. However, diuretics have no effect on how much fat you have. They just make you lose water from your body. They should never be used as a way to lose weight. They can be harmful because they take important minerals from your body.

3) Gimmicks are dangerous.
There are many gimmicks which are supposed to help you lose weight. There are wraps, and saunas, and machines that are supposed to shake the fat off you.

These gimmicks don't work. They don't make your body use up fat. Some of them make you lose some water from your body. After you lose water, you will weigh a little less. However, your body will soon replace the water it has lost. You will not end up any thinner.

The only people who benefit from these gimmicks are the people who make them and sell them.

4) Meal Replacement Drinks are dangerous.
These drinks are expensive and they usually don't work well. Many of them do not give you all the different foods your body needs.

If you use one of these drinks, don't take it for more than 10 days in any month. For the rest of the month, eat good food.

Learn to eat different foods rather than to depend on these drinks.

5) Operations are dangerous.

Some women who are desperate to lose weight have operations. Some women have some of their fat carved away or suctioned out. Others have part of their stomachs stapled closed. Some women have part of their intestines removed so that their food is not all absorbed. Others even have their jaws wired shut to prevent them from eating!

These are very dangerous and unnecessary operations. Many women have died after having them. They are not the way to choose to lose weight.

6) Eating disorders are dangerous.

Anorexia and Bulimia are called "eating disorders". People who have anorexia or bulimia are terrified of being fat.

Anorexia.

Most people with anorexia are young women between 13 and 30. Women with anorexia starve themselves until they become extremely thin and very sick. Sometimes they weigh only 80 or 90 pounds, but they still think they are fat. Because they eat so little, they become very tired. Their heart rates may be very slow, and they may not have menstrual periods.

Anorexia is a very serious condition. One out of every seven women who have it die of it.

Bulimia.
People with bulimia try to control their weight a different way. First they eat a great deal of food. Then they get rid of the food by either making themselves throw up, or by using laxatives, or by fasting, or by doing lots of exercise.

Bulimia is also very dangerous to your health. Bulimia can cause stomach problems, seizures, dental problems, and kidney damage. It can also kill you.

If you know someone with an extreme fear of gaining weight, talk to her about anorexia and bulimia. If you think your friend needs help, get her to talk with a doctor or a nutritionist who knows about eating disorders. She might also be able to join a support group for people with eating disorders.

Remember, most people with eating disorders don't think they are in danger. Even if your friend insists that she doesn't have a problem, don't stop. Give her some information and the phone number of someone who could help her.

How to quit smoking without gaining weight.

Smoking is clearly bad for your health. However, many women who smoke are afraid to quit smoking. This is because they are afraid they will gain weight. But, this does not always happen. Many people quit smoking and don't gain any weight at all.

Here are some ideas to help you quit smoking without gaining weight:

- Don't replace your after-dinner cigarette with a big dessert.
- If you are used to having something in your mouth, try sugarless candy or gum.
- If you want to eat something, eat raw fruit or vegetables or cheese.
- Drink lots of water.
- Keep your hands busy while you are watching TV. Do puzzles, or knit, or exercise. Do whatever you enjoy, but don't eat instead of smoking.
- Most people who smoke want a cigarette when they are upset. If this happens when you are upset, don't eat instead of smoking. Go for a walk, or call a friend.

After a few weeks, the craving for cigarettes will be much less. So will your craving for food. So, don't keep on harming yourself by smoking because you are afraid of gaining weight.

Give yourself a break. Don't be controlled by how you look. Don't put things off until you are thin, or until you think that you look "perfect".

If you do want to lose weight, forget about "going on a diet". You need a long-lasting way of losing weight and keeping it off. The best way to lose extra fat is to:

- eat only healthy food, and
- start being more active.

Do this, and you'll feel better. You will lose extra fat, and gaining weight won't be a problem any more.

Over-The-Counter Drugs

6

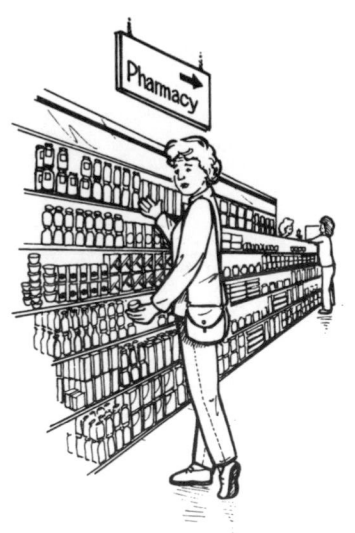

OVER-THE-COUNTER DRUGS

Over-the-counter drugs are medicines that you can buy without a prescription. Aspirin, cough medicines, decongestants and laxatives are over-the-counter drugs.

Over-the-counter drugs are a cheap and easy way to handle minor problems, such as coughs or headaches. However, even though you can buy them without a prescription, they are still powerful drugs. Like any drug, they can seriously hurt you if you don't use them properly.

Before you take any drug, remember the following rules:

Rules for using over-the-counter drugs safely:

1) Only take drugs when you are sure you need them.

2) Talk with your druggist to find out if the drug is safe for you.

This is very important because some drugs are not safe for some people. Go ahead and talk with your druggist. Part of his or her job is to help people. Ask for help, and be on the safe side.

- Tell your druggist about the **health problem** you are buying the drug for.
- Tell your druggist about any **other health problems** you have, such as diabetes or high blood pressure.
- Tell your druggist if you think you are **pregnant**. If so, don't take any drugs until you are sure they are safe.
- Tell your druggist about **any other drugs** you are taking. Mention both prescription and over-the-counter drugs. Remember to mention birth control pills and vitamins. Do this even if you can't see any connection between these drugs and your present problem.
- Tell your druggist about **any allergies** you may have.

3) Talk with your druggist about how to take the drug.

- Find out how and when to take the drug. (This is called the "dosage".)
- Find out what you can eat while taking this drug. Find out if you should take the drug before you eat, after you eat, or on an empty stomach.
- Find out if the drug will make you too sleepy to do things like drive a car.
- Find out if you can drink alcohol while taking the drug.
- If you think you may forget your instructions, ask the druggist to write them down for you.

4) Only take over-the-counter drugs for 2 to 3 days. If your problem is still there after 2 or 3 days, then call your doctor.

5) Follow directions carefully.
Before you take your medicine, carefully read the label or the instructions. When you are sure about what you should do, follow the directions. If you don't understand them, ask your druggist.

6) **Store your drugs carefully.**

Always keep your drugs in the container they came in. Then all the instructions will be on the label. The label should tell you if the drug must be kept cool or not. **Always store medicines out of the reach of children!**

7) **Call your doctor or your druggist if you get any unusual side effects.**

Side effects are extra ways that a drug affects you. These are different from the effect that the drug is supposed to have. Some common side effects are headaches, drowsiness, dizziness, irregular heartbeats, rashes, nausea, diarrhea, and constipation. Your doctor or druggist should warn you about which side effects to expect. Some side effects are only annoying, but some are dangerous. If you have any side effects or problems which no one warned you about, call your doctor.

8) Always carry a list of all the drugs you are taking.

Also carry a list of any drugs you are allergic to.

Remember, you can buy generic drugs. Generic drugs are sometimes called "no-name drugs". They are often sold as the "store brand". They have the same chemicals in them as brand name drugs, but they are cheaper. If you are not sure what to buy, get advice.

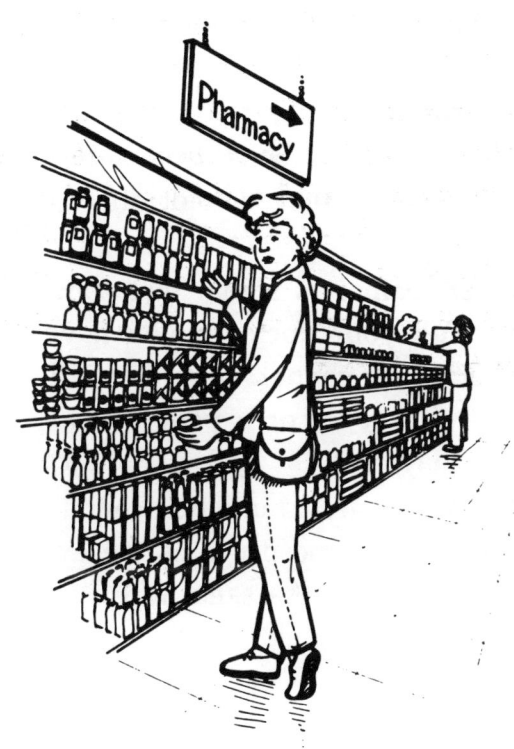

Pain Pills

"What are they good for?"

- Most over-the-counter pain pills contain either the drug ASA (aspirin) or the drug acetaminophen (Tylenol). They are very good drugs for fever and for minor pains such as headaches.

- Aspirin is very useful for arthritis. However, check with your doctor before you start taking aspirin regularly.

- Don't take aspirin if you have an ulcer.

"How do they work?"

- Pain pills stop your body from feeling pain for a while. However, they do not affect the cause of your pain.

- Remember: pain is a signal that something is wrong. Call your doctor if you have a fever or a pain which you cannot explain. Call your doctor if you have a fever or a pain which lasts longer than two days.

- Plain ASA and acetaminophen contain smaller amounts of the same drugs as the extra-strength kinds. They work the same way and they are often much cheaper.

"How can I use them safely?"

We use aspirin so often that we can forget that it is a powerful drug. So be careful!

* Keep all aspirin and acetaminophen away from children. Aspirin is the number one cause of poisoning in children. Be very careful with the flavoured ones which children like.

* Aspirin can be dangerous when you have a virus. If you or your child has a fever caused by a virus, do not take aspirin. Colds, flu, measles, mumps and chicken pox are all caused by a virus. Acetaminophen is much safer than aspirin for people with these diseases.

* Avoid taking ASA or any drug in the first three months of your pregnancy. Also avoid ASA in the last months of your pregnancy.

"What could I do besides use this drug?"

* Often a rest and something to eat or drink will help a minor headache.

* Sit or lie down, relax, and close your eyes. Breathe deeply and slowly.

* If you have a headache or a fever due to a cold, give your body a rest.

* If you often get headaches, especially when you first wake up, see your doctor. These headaches could mean that you have a more serious illness.

Menstrual Pain Drugs

"What are they good for?"

- Menstrual pain medicines can be used for pain before and during your menstrual period.
- If you have severe pain, these medicines are not strong enough.

"How do they work?"

- They contain several ingredients. The only useful ingredient is the aspirin or acetaminophen for the pain. The other ingredients are not very useful for menstrual pain.

"How can I use them safely?"

- Most menstrual pain can be relieved by taking plain aspirin or acetaminophen. Aspirin and acetaminophen are much cheaper by themselves than when they are combined with these other useless drugs.
- Most menstrual pain relievers contain aspirin or acetaminophen. Aspirin can be very dangerous for some people at some times. Please read p. 177 on how to use aspirin safely.
- If you have the flu, don't take menstrual pain relievers which contain aspirin. Please read p. 177.

"What could I do besides use this drug?"

- Eat good food and exercise regularly, especially in the week before your period is due.
- Drink plenty of water and eat very little salt in the week before your period.
- If you have severe menstrual pain, talk with your doctor. You will need a stronger drug than these over-the-counter pills. Your doctor may give you an "anti-prostaglandin" drug.

Antacids

"What are they good for?"

- Antacids are very helpful for heartburn and ulcers.
- They are not very useful for indigestion, nausea, upset stomachs, or gas.

"How do they work?"

- You have a strong acid in your stomach which digests your food. This acid doesn't burn your stomach because your stomach has a lining which protects it.
- Your esophagus is the tube which brings food down to your stomach. If some of the stomach acid gets up into your esophagus, it hurts. This is because the esophagus doesn't have a lining to protect it. This pain is called "heartburn". Antacids cut down the amount of acid in your stomach. That is why they are useful for heartburn.
- Stomach acid also causes pain if you have an ulcer. Ulcers are open sores inside your stomach. Ulcers hurt more when they are covered in stomach acid. Because antacids reduce the amount of acid in your stomach, they are very useful for ulcers.

"How can I use them safely?"

- Don't take antacids for a long time. This is why:
  - Antacids reduce the amount of acid in your stomach. You need this acid to digest your food. If you use antacids for a long time, your food won't be digested properly. You will end up with indigestion, diarrhea or constipation.
  - Antacids can cover up a serious problem, such as cancer of the stomach.
- Some antacids contain a lot of sodium. If you need to avoid salt, then you need to avoid these antacids. Read the labels, or ask your druggist.
- People with certain diseases must not take antacids. Check with your doctor or druggist.

"What could I do besides use this drug?"

- If you often have heartburn, stop drinking coffee and don't lie down after meals. Eating smaller meals will also help.
- If you have indigestion, antacids will not help you much. Indigestion can be caused by some kinds of foods and medicines. It can also be caused by smoking and by stress. However, indigestion is often caused by eating or drinking - too much or too fast. You can often get rid of your indigestion by changing what you eat and how you eat.
- If you often have heartburn or indigestion, see your doctor.

Laxatives

"What are they good for?"

- Laxatives relieve constipation. You are constipated when you have hard, dry bowel movements. You are not constipated just because you don't have a bowel movement every day.
- Laxatives can be used now and again. However, laxatives should not be used regularly.
- Laxatives are not meant for children.

"How do they work?"

They work three ways:
- by softening the contents of your bowel, or
- by adding bulk (solids) to the contents of your bowel, or
- by making your bowel more active.

"How can I use them safely?"

- Before you use a laxative, try eating more foods which contain fibre.
- Use mild, slow-acting laxatives. Fast-acting, strong laxatives can cause painful cramps and diarrhea.
- Pregnant women should only use slow-acting laxatives.
- Laxatives should not be used regularly. If you are constipated often, check with your doctor.

"What could I do besides use this drug?"

- Usually constipation is caused by what you eat. To prevent constipation, eat more foods which contain fibre, such as cereals, grains, fruits and vegetables.
- Drink more water and more fruit juice.
- Be more active. Exercise helps constipation.

Anti-Diarrhea Medicines

"What are they good for?"

- These medicines are for simple diarrhea.
- If your baby or child has diarrhea, check with your doctor. Talk with your doctor before you give them this kind of medicine. In the meantime, give them clear liquids such as water, broth, or Jello. Do not give them milk products at this time.

"How do they work?"

- Anti-diarrhea medicines make the contents of your bowel more solid.
- Some of them also pick up some of the poisons which may have caused the diarrhea.
- Stronger ones stop your bowel from moving for a while.

"How can I use them safely?"

- Don't use anti-diarrhea medicines for very long. If your diarrhea doesn't go away after a few days, call your doctor.
- If you have diarrhea along with cramps, fever, or vomiting, call your doctor.
- Do not give anti-diarrhea medicines to children without checking with your doctor.

"What could I do besides use this drug?"

- Diarrhea can be caused by something bad in your food or water, by infection, or by stress. Most diarrhea goes away on its own in a couple days without drugs.

- Before using an anti-diarrhea medicine, try drinking lots of clear fluids, like water, tea or broth. Then try easy-to-digest foods such as plain yogurt, bananas, poached eggs, or rice.

- Some people get diarrhea when they take antibiotics. Yogurt may help to prevent this kind of diarrhea.

Cough Medicines

"What are they good for?"

- Cough medicines make you cough less. This is not always a good thing. Not all coughs should be stopped.
- A cough is useful if it brings up mucus (thick fluid) from your lungs. This is called a "productive" cough. You should not try to stop it.
- A cough is not useful if it doesn't bring up any mucus. This is called a "dry" cough. It will make your throat sore, and it will keep you awake. It's OK to try to stop this kind of cough.
- For dry coughs, a prescription cough medicine works much better than any over-the-counter brand.

"How do they work?"

- There are different kinds of cough medicine.
- Some cough medicines contains a drug which affects the cough control centre in your brain. This kind is called a "cough suppressant".
- Other cough medicines contain a drug which thins the mucus in your nose and lungs. This kind is called an "expectorant".
- Many cough medicines contain both a suppressant and an expectorant. These are not very useful because the suppressant and the expectorant work against each other.

- Choose the kind of cough medicine which does what you need it to do.

"How can I use them safely?"
- Most coughs are caused by colds. They go away soon after your cold is better.
- Some coughs are more serious.
  - Call your doctor if you have a cough and severe chest pains, or shortness of breath.
  - Call your doctor if your cough produces mucus with blood in it.
  - Call your doctor if you have a cough and fever for 2 or 3 days.
  - Call your doctor if your cough lasts longer than your cold.
- Before you choose a cough medicine, check with your druggist to make sure it is safe for you.

"What could I do besides use this drug?"
- Give your body a rest when you are sick.
- Keep the air in your house moist with a vaporizer, or a kettle set on low for a while. Moisture often works as well as medicine.
- Drink plenty of fluids, such as tea, juice, or water.
- Cut down on your own smoking, and the smoking in your house.
- Try a hot drink of water, honey and lemon juice.

Cold Medicines

"What are they good for?"

- Cold medicines do not cure colds. Colds are caused by viruses, and there are no drugs which can kill viruses. Whether you take a "cold remedy" or not, it usually takes about seven days to get rid of a virus.
- Cold medicines work on some of the cold symptoms.

"How do they work?"

Cold medicines usually contain several ingredients:

- ASA or acetaminophen for your pain and fever,
- cough medicine to stop you from coughing,
- decongestants, which may help to open up your nasal passages,
- antihistamines, which dry up your nose and may make your cough worse.

(Cold medicines do not contain antibiotics because antibiotics are useless for colds.)

"How can I use them safely?"

- Check with your doctor or your druggist to see if the drug is safe for you. Ask your doctor or druggist if the drug will be useful for you.
- Do not drink alcohol when taking a cold medicine. Together they make you very drowsy.
- Do not use nose sprays for more than 3 days at a time. If you take them for very long, they can make your nose more congested instead of less.
- Cold medicines are not good for children.
- Do not take cold medicines when you are pregnant.
- If you use a cold medicine, choose the kind which treats only one symptom. Ask your druggist if you aren't sure.

"What could I do besides use this drug?"

- Give your body a rest when you have a cold.
- Eat well, and drink plenty of fluids, especially fruit juices.
- Avoid alcohol.
- Cut down on smoking.
- Keep the air in your house moist with a vaporizer, or a kettle set on low for a while.

Antihistamines

"What are they good for?"

- Antihistamines can relieve the symptoms of allergies, such as hay fever and hives. They cannot cure allergies.
- Some antihistamines help to control the nausea caused by travel sickness.
- They cannot cure colds, and they should not be used for colds.
- They are not useful for asthma.

"How do they work?"

- Some of them can help to dry up runny eyes and noses which are caused by allergies.
- Some of them help stop the itch from rashes caused by allergies.

"How can I use them safely?"

- Antihistamines are not safe for everyone. Check with your druggist before you buy one.
- They have many side effects. A very common one is drowsiness. You should not take them if you are going to be driving, or if you need to stay awake.
- Don't take them with sleeping pills or with alcohol. Together they can make you very sleepy.

"What could I do besides use this drug?"

- It may be very hard to avoid the thing you are allergic to. If your allergy bothers you a lot, or lasts for a long time, see your doctor.

You and
Your Doctor

7

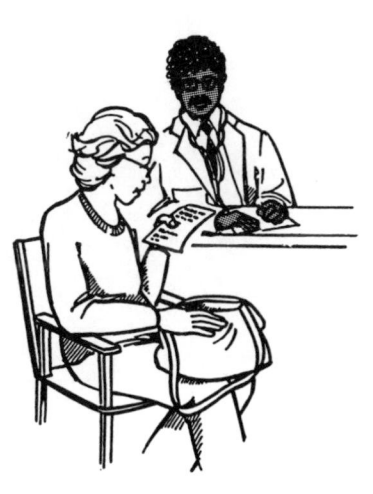

YOU AND YOUR DOCTOR

This chapter contains information about how to
deal with doctors and other medical people. It
gives you information about your rights and your
responsibilities as a patient.

You may not need this information right now.
However, the next time you go to a doctor, or to a
hospital, you might need to know what this
chapter says. Look over the list of topics in the
Table of Contents, or look through the chapter.
Then you'll know where to find the information
when you need it.

Your Rights and Responsibilities as a Patient.

The most important things to remember about being
a patient are:

1. Your body belongs to you. You have the right
to decide what happens to it.

2. Your doctor's job is to help you take care of
yourself.

When you are dealing with your doctor, you have
the right to know what is going on. You have the
right to ask questions, and the right to get answers.

This may be easier said than done. It is easy to feel confused and afraid when you are dealing with doctors and people in hospitals. Sometimes they talk to you in words that you don't understand. Sometimes they tell you to do things without telling you why. Sometimes they give you medicine without giving you enough information about it.

If this ever happens to you, you need to remember that you have both rights and responsibilities as a patient. You have the responsibility to ask the questions which you need to ask. You also have a right to get answers. If you are confused or afraid about your treatment, that's a sign that you need to ask more questions. If you are confused or afraid about your treatment, your doctor needs to give you more answers.

Asking questions is the first step in starting to work with your doctor. If you work with your doctor, you can solve your health problems together.

Your Rights as a Patient.

Patients have both legal and moral (or human) rights.

Most of your rights are legal rights. Legal rights are yours by law. This means that doctors and nurses **must** give you these rights as a patient.

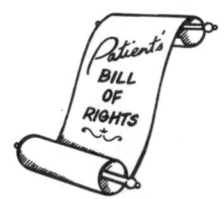

Some rights are moral rights. These are rights which doctors and nurses have promised to give to their patients. In other words, doctors and nurses **should** give these rights to their patients. There rights are usually covered by the nurses' and doctors' "Code of Ethics".

Legal Rights.

When you are a patient, you have these legal rights:
1. You have the right to a **good standard of care**.

2. You have the right to **full information** about your illness in words that you can understand. This means that you have the right to understand the treatment you are being given. You have the right to understand what you are signing before you sign it. You have the right to know the names and jobs of anyone who is taking care of you.

3. You have the right to **refuse a treatment**. This is always true unless you have certain serious infections, such as gonorrhea and tuberculosis. You must accept treatment for these diseases because they are serious, and they can be spread to others.

4. You have the right to **agree** to your **treatment**. (You may be asked to show that you agree by signing a "consent form".)

5. You have the right to **privacy**. Your files and any information about you is confidential. This means that this information can only be given to someone else if you give permission. This is called the right to confidentiality.

6. You have the right to **refuse** to be in **experiments**, for research or for teaching.

7. You have the right to be treated with **respect**. This is true no matter what your sex, or your race, or your colour is. This is true no matter what your religion, your schooling, your income, or your life-style is.

8. You have the right to **choose** your own doctor. (This includes the right to change doctors. However, it is much better to build a good relationship with one doctor, than to change doctors over and over.)

9. You have the right to be treated in an **emergency**.

Moral Rights.

When you are a patient, you have these moral rights:

1. You have the right to be treated with respect and dignity.

2. You have the right to get a second opinion from another doctor if you want one.

3. You have the right to have your relatives respected during your stay in hospital.

4. You have the right to die with dignity. This means that, when you are dying, you and your family can decide what type of care you will get.

Rights of Patients with Mental Health Problems

Each province has laws which cover the rights of patients with mental health problems. These rights are not the same across the country. In some provinces, mental patients have more rights than in others. For example, it is much easier to have control over your treatment in some provinces than in others.

If you have any questions, talk with someone at the Canadian Mental Health Association. You could also talk with a lawyer, or with a Patient Advocate. Some hospitals now have Patient Advocates. They speak for the rights of patients.

How to complain if you think your rights have been ignored.

If you think your rights have been ignored, you can take these steps. Start with number 1. If you are not happy with the response you get, go on to the next step.

1. Talk with the doctor or health worker whom you are upset with.

2. Talk with the supervisor of the person whom you are upset with.

3. Write a letter to the administrator of the hospital.

4. Write to the professional organization which the person belongs to. Doctors belong to a provincial College of Physicians and Surgeons. Nurses belong to a provincial College of Nurses.

5. Talk with a Patients' Rights Association.

6. Talk with a lawyer who has experience with health laws. You could call Legal Aid to see if they could help you.

Your Responsibilities as a Patient.

If you want more control over your health, then you will also have to take on more responsibility. Power and responsibility go together. When you are a patient, you have these responsibilities:

1. You have the responsibility to take care of yourself. To take good care of yourself, you need good information. You need to find out all you can about your treatments and your drugs.

2. You have the responsibility to tell all your symptoms to the people taking care of you. Talk with them about all the things you are worried about. You can't expect people to read your mind.

3. You have the responsibility to follow instructions after you have agreed to them. This does not mean that you cannot stop your treatment at any time. However, don't start a treatment if you are not planning to carry on with it.

4. You have the responsibility to treat health care workers with the same respect that you expect.

Being responsible for your health means being an active patient. Ask questions, and find out as much as you can. Make decisions about your health with your doctor. In the end, your doctor will be helping you to take care of yourself.

How to choose a doctor.

If you want to be an active patient, you will need to find a good doctor. You will need to find one that you like and trust. This may take you some time. The best time to look for a doctor is when you are well. Don't wait until you or your family are sick!

One way to find a good doctor is to ask other people about their doctors. Check with your friends, and with the people you work with. Ask your public health nurse too. Then, when you have a few names, call the doctors' offices and ask some questions.

These questions might help you choose:

1. Does the doctor take new patients?
2. Is the doctor a man or a woman?
3. Will the doctor take my whole family as patients?
4. How long will I have to wait to get an appointment?
5. How long do patients have to wait in the waiting room?

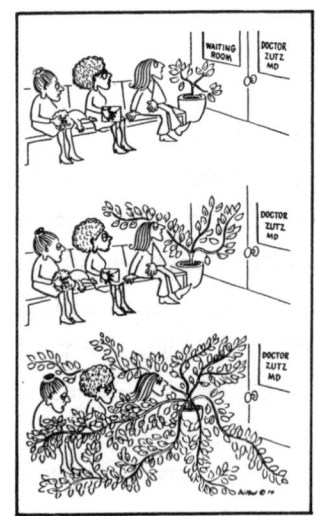

© Bulbul, 1974

6. Is the doctor's office near a laboratory in case I have to have x-rays or blood tests?
7. Is the doctor paid by the medical plan in this province? If not, how much will an appointment cost? Will I be charged any extra "administrative" fees?
8. Does the doctor charge more than the medical plan will pay for? How much more?
9. What are the doctor's office hours?
10. Will I always be able to see my doctor? Or, will I often see student doctors or other doctors in the same office?
11. Who will see me if I get sick at night or on the week-ends?
12. Does the doctor make house calls?
13. Which hospital does the doctor work at?

Before your first visit, think about the kind of person you want your doctor to be. Is it important that your doctor is a friendly, kind person? Do you want someone who will answer all your questions? Do you want someone who takes charge? Do you want a doctor who discusses your problem with you so together you can decide what to do?

Then, at the visit, you can see if this doctor seems like the right doctor for you. You may also have other questions for him or her. For example, you may want to know if she gives hormones to women during menopause. Or, you may want to know if he approves of natural childbirth. You may also want to know what this doctor thinks about women who ask a lot of questions!!

This may seem like a lot of work. However, it's worth it to find a doctor you like. And, remember. If you aren't happy with your new doctor, you have the right to complain. You have the right to ask for what you want. If this doesn't work, you have the right to leave that doctor and find one you do like.

"It's too much trouble. It's easier to just go to Emergency."

Why a family doctor is better than the Emergency Department:

Many people don't have a family doctor. Instead they go to the Emergency Department in a hospital when they are sick.

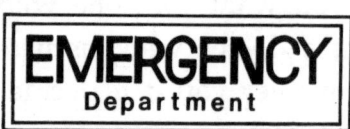

This is <u>not</u> a good idea.

Here's why:

- **The Emergency Department is only for real emergencies.**
  It should be left free for those who really need it.
- **The Emergency Department is not set up to deal with smaller problems.**
  The nurses and doctors don't have much time to talk with you. They don't have time to talk about what caused your problem. They don't have time to talk about how you could prevent it from happening again. They don't have time to talk about your other health problems. They only have time to give you something to help you right then.
  For example, you may have a bad headache. They will likely give you pain pills. However, they won't have time to discuss the reasons for your headache, or how to prevent another one. Pills are a short-term answer. What we really need are long-term answers to our health problems.
- **You may see a different nurse and doctor every time you go.**
  They won't know you, and they won't have your full medical history.
- **If your problem needs to be checked again, the hospital doctor will send you to your family doctor for a check-up anyway.**

Don't use the Emergency Department instead of a family doctor. You can get much better care if you get to know a good family doctor.

If you have a medical problem which you are worried about, night or day, call your doctor. At night, their answering service will get someone to call you. Together you can decide what to do.

Preparing for a doctor's appointment.

When you need to go to the doctor, it is a good idea to prepare for your appointment. While you are still at home, think about your problem. Be ready to describe your problem as clearly as you can.

1. Make a written list of all your symptoms.
Write down anything which you think seems different. For example, you might write down:

"pain in my stomach, no appetite, tired all the time".

2. Describe your problem.
Try to describe your problem as well as you can. Think about how long it has been going on. Think about whether it has been getting better or worse. Think about what makes you feel better. For example, drinking milk may help your stomach pain. Then try to remember what makes you feel worse. Perhaps eating spicy food makes your stomach pain worse.

3. Think about what medicines you are taking.
Your doctor needs to know about all your prescription drugs, such as antibiotics and birth control pills. Your doctor also needs to know about any medicines you buy for yourself, such as aspirin and vitamin pills. Your doctor needs to know the exact names of the medicines, and how long you have been taking each one.

4. Think about whether you could be pregnant.
If you might be pregnant, tell your doctor. There are some medicines and tests which you must not have if you are pregnant.
If you might be pregnant, tell your doctor. If you are breast-feeding, tell your doctor. Some medicines must not be taken by breast-feeding women.

5. Think about what medical tests you have had lately.
X-rays and blood tests are common medical tests. These tests usually do not need to be repeated if they were done recently.

6. Write down any questions you want to ask the doctor.
If you don't write your questions down, it is very easy to forget them. Be sure you put these two questions on your list: *"Why am I sick?"* and *"What can I do so I won't get sick again?"*

Even if your questions seem foolish to you, go ahead and ask them! You have the right to ask. Many doctors like patients who want to be involved in their health care. If your doctor never pays attention to your questions, point this out to her or him. If your doctor is always too busy to answer your questions, you may need to find a new doctor.

7. Think about what you want from your doctor. This is very important to think about. You may want a diagnosis, or you may want some medicine. Or, you may want advice, or comfort, or all of these things. If you know what you want, you have a much better chance of getting it.

If you are sick or worried, all of this thinking and planning may be a big chore. However, planning really helps. If you are well prepared, you will get better results. You and your doctor will have a much better chance of figuring out what is wrong with you.

At the Appointment.

Usually, the doctor will want to do two things:
1. Talk with you to get your medical history.
2. Examine you to try to see what's wrong with you.

Your medical history.

Your doctor needs to talk with you to get your "medical history". Your doctor will likely ask you about your present sickness, your past health, and your personal life.

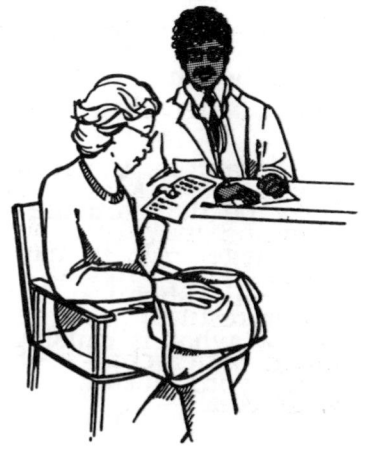

1. When the doctor asks you about your present sickness, use your list of symptoms to help you. Let your doctor know that you have spent some time thinking about your problem. Let the doctor know why you think something is wrong. Your doctor may also ask you how your sickness is affecting other parts of your body. This will help you and the doctor understand the sickness better.

2. The doctor will want to know about **your past health**. The doctor should find out about sicknesses and operations you have had. Your doctor should ask you about what medicines you are taking, and how they affect you. Your doctor will also ask if you have had any bad or allergic reactions to any medicine. She or he will also likely ask about your family's health.

3. The doctor will likely ask you some questions about **your personal life**. These questions can give some very important information about you and your health.

For example, the reason for your stomach trouble may be that you are very worried about your marriage. Or, it may be that you are working with a certain chemical at your job. If you think you know what is causing your problem, talk it over with your doctor.

Your doctor may also ask you about what you eat, and if you drink, or smoke, or use illegal drugs. Your doctor may also ask you about the amount of stress in your life. Stress can cause many health problems. (If you want some more information on Stress, please read Chapter 2, <u>Dealing With Your "Nerves"</u>.)

If your doctor forgets to ask you about something which you think is important, go ahead and mention it. You know your own body best.

The more you can tell your doctor about your health problem, the better. The more you can find out about your health care, the better. If you ask questions, you might be able to avoid an operation. If you ask questions, you might be able to avoid an expensive medicine, or a dangerous medicine. Talking things over with your doctor could save your life.

Your physical examination.
Next, your doctor will usually give you a physical examination. During the examination, you have a right to know what the doctor is doing and why. If you don't understand what's going on, ask! If you are nervous about going to the doctor, you could take a friend along for support.

Most parts of this examination should not hurt. If they do, let the doctor know. It might be because of your sickness, or because you are very nervous. It could also be that the doctor needs to be a little more careful.

Before you leave, you should know what the doctor thinks is wrong with you. This is called the diagnosis. You should know the medical name for your illness. You should know how and why you got sick, and how to prevent it in the future.

If your doctor thinks that you need treatment, you should know what kind it will be. You should also know how well this treatment might work.

Treatment for your health problem.

In this section, you will find some information on
• medical tests,
• using medicine safely,
• coping in the hospital.

Medical tests.

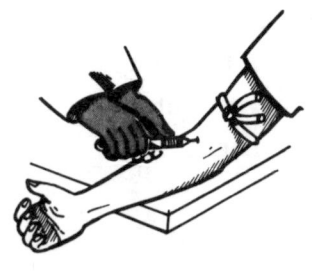

The doctor may send you to have some tests, such as x-rays or blood tests. You have the right to know why these tests are being done, and how important they are. Some tests do not have to be repeated if they were done recently. However, sometimes it is helpful to repeat tests to see if anything has changed.

When the test results come back, the doctor will let you know if there is a problem. You can also phone and ask for the results. If you don't understand what they mean, ask until you do. If you do not hear back about your tests, it likely means that they were normal.

Using medicine safely.

Medicines can be very powerful. They can help you, but they can also seriously hurt you. Before you take any medicine, find out if it is safe for you.

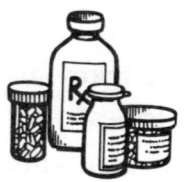

1. **Don't use medicine unless you really need it.** There are many kinds of medicine which you don't need. For minor problems, medicine can never take the place of good food and exercise. For example, exercise is a much better way to deal with sleeping problems than sleeping pills. And headaches often go away after a cup of tea and a rest.

When your doctor suggests a medicine, ask if there is anything else you could do for your problem. Don't expect to get some medicine every time you go to your doctor. Doctors sometimes give medicine only because they think you want it. Be sure you really need a medicine before you take it.

2. Find out as much as you can about your medicines.

Here are some questions to ask:

- What is the name of the medicine?
- What is the medicine supposed to do for me?
- How much should I take, and how often should I take it? ("This is called the "dosage".)
- How long should I take it?
- How should I take it? Should I take it with milk or water? Should I take it with meals or not?
- Can I take this medicine if I am taking other medicines?
- What side effects does this medicine have? What should I do if they happen? (Side effects are extra ways that a drug affects you. These are different from the effects the drug is supposed to have.)
- What foods or drinks should I avoid when I am taking this medicine? What about alcohol?
- What activities should I avoid when I am taking this medicine? For example, can I drive my car? Can I continue to work?
- Can I take this medicine if I am pregnant?
- Can I take this medicine if I am breast-feeding?
- Can I buy it as a no-name or generic drug?
- Have other patients of yours used this medicine before, or is this a new, experimental drug?

Go ahead and ask these questions. Doctors are not perfect. Sometimes they make mistakes, and sometimes they forget important things.

You may want to write down the information about how to take your new medicine. This will help you remember. If you want to, you can always ask your druggist questions too. Druggists are often very helpful. When you pick up your prescription, make sure the label is clear. Make sure you can read the instructions.

3. Follow directions carefully.
Take your medicine exactly as you have been told to. Before you take your medicine, read the label carefully. Then put the medicine down. Then pick it up and read the label again. When you are sure about what you should do, follow the directions.

Don't take any more or any less than your doctor has told you to take. Serious problems can happen if you do. Never take your medicine in the dark; it's easy to make mistakes. If you have a poor memory, you may need a system to help you remember when to take your medicine.

And if you are taking an antibiotic, be sure to finish the prescription.

4. Don't share medicines.

Don't take any of your friend's medicines, and don't give your medicine to your friends. You can do more harm than good. What is good for one person can kill another.

5. Store your prescriptions carefully.

Storing your medicines properly is very important. Some should be kept cool and some should not. If you aren't sure, ask your druggist.

If you have old medicine, don't use it until you check the expiry date. The expiry date tells you when it is no longer good. (This is a good reason for keeping all medicines in the bottles they came in. Then all the important information should be on the label.)

> Store all your medicine in a place children cannot reach. Aspirin is the number one cause of poisoning in children!

6. **Ask for the least expensive brand of medicine.**
Generic drugs (or no-name drugs) are usually the
cheapest kind. They contain the same chemicals so
they are usually just as good.

If you are on a Drug Plan, your prescriptions will be
paid for. If you get a prescription which is not
covered by the Plan, let your doctor know. She or
he may be able to change the prescription. If not,
they may be able to arrange things so you won't
have to pay.

7. **Pay attention to how the medicine affects you.**
Side effects are extra ways that a drug affects you.
Side effects are different from the effect the drug is
supposed to have. Some common side effects are
headaches, drowsiness, dizziness, irregular
heartbeats, rashes, nausea, diarrhea, constipation, and
dry mouth.

Your doctor or druggist should warn you about
which side effects to expect. They should also tell
you how to deal with them. If you have any side
effects or problems which they didn't warn you
about, tell your doctor.

8. **Carry your important medical information with you.** Carry your medical facts in your wallet. If you have a special medical problem, always wear a medic-alert bracelet or necklace.

You should carry these important medical facts with you:
- the name and phone number of your doctor.
- the names of all the medicines you are taking.
- the names of any important health condition you have; such as diabetes, heart disease, pregnancy.
- the names of any allergies you may have.

Antibiotics

Antibiotics, such as penicillin, are very useful medicines because they fight infections. Because they are so useful, they are very popular. In fact antibiotics are so popular that many people take too many of them. As with any medicine, you should only take an antibiotic when you really need it.

Antibiotics only fight certain kinds of infections. An infection happens when bacteria or viruses grow in large amounts. Antibiotics can only kill bacteria, so they can only fight infections which are caused by bacteria. Antibiotics cannot kill viruses, so they cannot fight infections caused by viruses.

Strep throat and ear infections are caused by bacteria, so antibiotics are useful for these infections.

Colds and flus are caused by viruses, so antibiotics are <u>not</u> useful for colds and flus. Antibiotics are useless for an infection which is caused by a virus.

When you are taking antibiotics, you must finish the whole prescription. Here is why:

After two days of taking the antibiotic, you will usually feel much better. This is because the weakest bacteria will be dead by then.

However, the strongest bacteria are still alive. If you stop taking the antibiotic too soon, the strong bacteria can start to grow in larger numbers. This can become a serious infection. You can end up sicker than when you began. This is why you must take <u>all</u> the medicine, even after your symptoms are all gone. After you finish the full prescription, all the harmful bacteria should be killed.

For the same reason, you should never take some left-over antibiotic pills if you think you have an infection. If you need an antibiotic, see your doctor and get a full prescription.

Coping in the hospital.

If your doctor wants
you to have an
operation, think
about it carefully.
If it is not an
emergency, get a
second opinion from
a doctor who is not
a surgeon.

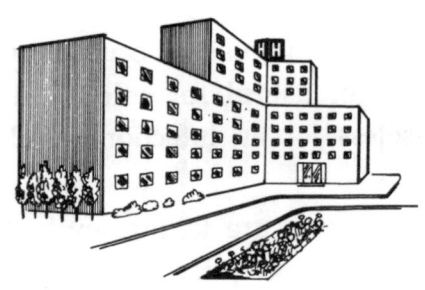

The answers to these questions might help you make
up your mind:
- What is my health problem called, in medical
  language?
- Is this operation necessary? What will happen to
  me if I don't have it? What other treatments
  could I have instead of an operation?
- Will this operation cure me entirely?
- Will I need another operation after this?
- What are the risks of the operation?
- What side effects can I expect from the operation?
- What other treatments will be needed?
- What exactly is going to be done to me?
- What medicines will be given to me, and what
  are their side effects?

- What tests will be done on me? for example: blood tests, x-rays, ECGs.
- Will I have a general anesthetic? (This is the kind that affects your whole body and makes you unconscious.) Or, will I have a local anesthetic? (This is the kind that only affects the part which is being operated on.)
- How long will I be in hospital?
- Will I need special equipment or services when I get home?
- Will I be well enough to care for my children when I get home?
- When will I be well enough to go back to work?

If you go into a hospital, your rights are the same as your rights in the doctor's office. You have the right to understand what is going on, and the right to be treated well. You can question anything which makes you uncomfortable.

If you have a problem in the hospital, ask for help. If you want to change something about your care, speak to your nurse. Perhaps you would like to take more or less medicine. Ask the nurse to speak with your doctor. If this doesn't work, you can ask your doctor yourself.

If someone asks you to sign some papers, read them carefully. If you don't understand what you are signing, ask someone to explain it to you. Some medicines affect how clearly you can think. Do not sign any important papers until you can think clearly.

There are many people working in hospitals. There are doctors, nurses, social workers, therapists, technicians, dieticians, chaplains, and maintenance staff. If you don't know who is treating you, you have the right to find out.

Some hospitals are called "teaching" hospitals. This means they train nurses, social workers, dieticians, and doctors. If you are in a teaching hospital, someone may want to examine you as part of their training. They must ask you for your permission before they ask you any questions. They must also ask you before they examine you. You may want to let them do this in order to help them learn. Or, you may want to refuse. It's up to you. You have the right to say "no"; many people do.

Sometimes doctors in training have a lot of time to talk with you, and to examine you. Sometimes these doctors pick up something which you or your doctor did not think of.

When you leave the hospital.

Some people need special care for a while after they leave the hospital. The social workers at the hospital can arrange this for you.

After you are discharged, you will need to know how to take care of yourself.

Here are some questions to ask before you leave the hospital:

- What were the results of my treatment?
- Do I need any other treatment?
- Do I need to see a doctor again? If so, who and when?
- How should I be feeling in the next couple of weeks? (This is important so you know if something is going wrong.)
- Which doctor should I contact if I am not feeling well? How do I contact this doctor?
- What medicine do I still need? Do I need a prescription?
- What supplies will I need? How and where do I get them?
- Do I need to follow a special diet?
- What exercise am I allowed to do?

If you get some of this information in writing, you may be able to remember it better.

Besides doctors, there are many other people who can help you with your health problems. You can also get help from these health workers:
- physiotherapists
- occupational therapists
- massage therapists
- chiropractors
- counsellors
- psychologists
- homeopaths
- acupuncturists
- Women's Health Centre workers

The public health nurses at your Health Unit can help you with many different health problems. They can also tell you about special clinics and groups and services in your area.

Here are some clinics and groups they could refer you to:
- prenatal classes
- baby clinics
- preschool services
- parenting groups
- mental health clinics
- dental services
- family planning clinics
- blood pressure clinics

When you deal with doctors or nurses or other medical workers, remember this. Their job is to help you take care of your health problems. The more you know about your health, the better you can work with your doctor. The more you know about your health, the better you can decide what is best for you.

After all, the most important person taking care of you is you!

Sex

8

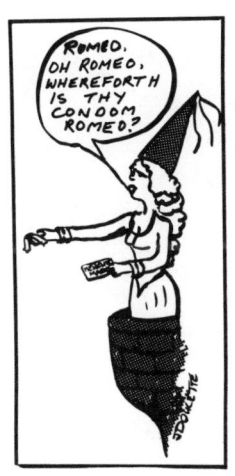

SEX

Sex can give you pleasure, but it can also cause worries and problems. One of the best ways to deal with your worries about sex is to find out as much as you can.

This is a long chapter. It deals with many things that people worry about. If you don't want to read the whole chapter, look over the list of topics in the Table of Contents, or look through the chapter. Find the sections which are interesting to you.

Sexual parts of your body.

Many of us don't know enough about the sexual parts of our bodies. We may not know what they look like. We may not know enough about what each part does. The more you know about your body and how it works, the better.

• The clitoris is the most sensitive part of your body. It is your sexual nerve centre. It is so sensitive that you may feel uncomfortable when it is touched directly.

You can only see a small part of your clitoris. The rest of it is under the skin under each of the inner lips. It almost reaches back to the opening of your vagina.

Your clitoris is a bit like a penis. It swells when it is excited. Your clitoris (not your vagina) produces orgasms. The only purpose of your clitoris is sexual pleasure.

Behind your clitoris, there are three openings: the urinary opening, the vaginal opening, and the anus. These openings are partly covered by outer and inner lips. These lips are called labia.

• The **urinary opening** is the opening where urine (or pee) comes out. It is very small and hard to see.

• The **vaginal opening** is the opening to your vagina. Your vagina leads to your uterus (or womb). Your vagina is where menstrual blood comes out. It is also the passage a baby comes through to be born.

Your vagina is <u>not</u> as sexually sensitive as your clitoris is. During sexual intercourse, the penis goes into the vagina. Semen is usually released in the vagina. (Semen is the liquid which comes out of a man's penis when he has an orgasm. Semen contains sperm, and a sperm can join with an egg to start a pregnancy.)

• The **anus** is the opening where bowel movements come out.

If you feel comfortable doing this, take a mirror and look at your sexual parts. (You will likely look a little different from the following picture. No two women look exactly the same.)

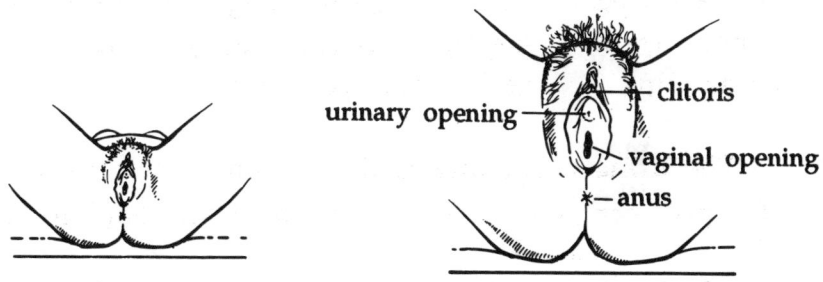

urinary opening — clitoris — vaginal opening — anus

You also have other sexual parts in your body. Touching your mouth, breasts, and ears can be exciting. Many people like touching and being touched all over their bodies.

Being "normal".

Many people worry about whether they have "normal" sex lives. When it comes to sex, it is hard to say what is "normal". Different people enjoy doing many different things.

For example:
- You may make love three times a day, or three times a month, or three times a year.
- You may have sex in many different positions, or just one.
- You may have orgasms in many positions, or just one.
- You may want an orgasm every time you make love.
- You may not care if you have an orgasm or not.

Each of these examples is "normal" and OK, if it is OK with you.

As long as no one gets hurt, and no one is forced to do anything, you don't have to worry about being "normal".

Your right to choose.

Sex is your choice. You have the right to choose who you make love with and when. You have the right to choose to make love with women or men. You have the right to choose if you want to make love or not. You have the right to say "yes" or "no" to anyone, anytime. You have the right to ask for sex, and the right to refuse it to someone else. You have the right to choose not to have any sexual partners. It's your choice.

Choosing is not always easy to do. Sometimes it is dangerous to insist on our right to choose. Some men, including our husbands, think they have a right to force us to have sex. They are wrong. They don't have the right.

Remember: you do not "owe" anyone sex. No matter how much money they spent, or how many dates you have been on, you don't owe anyone sex. You still have the right to choose.

Homosexuality.

If you are homosexual, then you are attracted to people of your own sex. If you are heterosexual, then you are attracted to people of the other sex. If you are bisexual, then you are attracted to people of both sexes.

Heterosexual people are often called "straight". Homosexual people are often called "gay". Many gay women prefer to be called "lesbians".

Some people worry about whether they are homosexual, and some people are frightened of homosexuals. If you are confused, here is some information which might help you:

- At least one out of every ten people is gay.
- It is not true that homosexual men are dangerous with children. In fact, most men who abuse children are heterosexuals.
- Lesbians and gay men are not sick. They are not sick and they don't need to be "cured".
- Lesbians and gay men have loving and caring relationships, the same as heterosexuals do.

You may be afraid of homosexuals because you are afraid of AIDS. This is a mistake for two reasons:
1. AIDS is not a disease which only homosexuals get. In many parts of the world, more heterosexuals than homosexuals have AIDS. Anyone who doesn't follow the rules of "Safer Sex" can get AIDS, whether they are straight or gay. (If you want to know more about AIDS and Safer Sex, please read p. 248 in this chapter.)
2. You cannot get AIDS in everyday situations. AIDS is not spread through air, water or food. AIDS is not spread by ordinary body contact, such as shaking hands. AIDS is nearly always spread during sex with an infected person. It also spread by sharing drug needles with an infected person.

It is not easy being gay in this culture. Most gay people have to hide the fact that they are gay. If they don't, they might lose their job, their children, and even their lives.

Although many straight people are confused and scared by gay people, many others are changing their attitudes. Many people now understand that homosexuality is not a sickness. Many people realize that they have nothing to fear from lesbians or gay men. Many people now believe that anyone can be a good worker, or a good parent, or a good friend, whether they are attracted to men or women.

If you want to find out more about homosexuality, you could talk with your public health nurse or with a doctor. You could talk with someone in the Planned Parenthood Association, or in the Canadian Mental Health Association. You could also talk with someone in a Gay Rights group.

Sexual problems.

Many problems with sex can be solved just by talking together. Talk with your partner as honestly and as carefully as you can.

You can't expect your partner to know what you like without telling him or her. Talk together about what you like and don't like about your sex life. Find out what your partner likes and doesn't like. These things change from time to time, so you may need to talk more than once.

For many people, the idea of talking is easier said than done. Sex is very difficult for many people to talk about because they are embarrassed.

Some men won't talk about sexual problems because they think that problems mean that they are not "good in bed". This is a mistake. Everyone has problems with sex sometimes.

Some women also believe that the man is in charge of sex. And, some women don't talk about sex because they find it very hard to ask for what they want. They don't ask for what they want, in bed or anywhere else.

You can change these ideas if you want to. If you start asking for what you want, then both of you could have an equal chance for a good sex life.

Some women don't talk about sex because they don't have words which they are comfortable using. They have words for sex that they use with their doctors, and words they use with their children. They also know slang sex words. However, many women don't like slang words because men often use them as angry, insulting words. They don't want to connect sex with anger and insults. The result is that these women don't talk much about sex.

If you are like these women, think about the words that you use. Talk with your partner about how you both feel about the words you use. If you realize that you don't like some words, you can change them. You and your partner may need to find other words which say what sex really means to you.

Even though it may be hard to do, talking about sex is very important. After all, sex is not just orgasms. Sex is a way that you show how you feel about each other. Talking can help you and your partner understand each other better, and this can help your sex life.

If talking together doesn't solve your problems, you may want to get help from someone else. You could talk with your public health nurse or your doctor. You could also talk with a sex therapist. Ask your public health nurse or your doctor to suggest some therapists to you. Many Family Counselling Services have counsellors who are trained in sex therapy.

Some women have problems with sex because they were sexually assaulted in the past. If you were sexually assaulted, you could talk about it with other women in a self-help group. You may also want to talk with a counsellor. Some counsellors have special training to help women who have been victims of sexual violence.

Interest in sex.

The people on TV shows seem to be interested in sex any time, and all the time. Most of us aren't like these people.

Some women are interested in sex a lot. Some are not interested very often at all. There is no rule that says how often you "should" want sex. However, you may have a problem if you are more interested or less interested than your partner is.

Many things can affect how interested you are in sex. Here are some of the those things:

Your Menstrual Cycle.

Many women say that their interest in sex changes a lot during their menstrual cycle. Some women are more interested before their periods. Some women are more interested during their periods, and others are not interested at all.

(There is no medical reason why you can't have sex during your period. However, some women don't like it because they don't feel well, or because they find it too messy).

Your Emotions.

Your emotions have a big effect on your interest in sex. If you are sick or tired or scared, you likely aren't as interested as when you are feeling good.

Painful Sex.

Intercourse should not hurt. But, there are some times when it does.

Here are some reasons why intercourse may hurt:
• Intercourse may hurt if you have a vaginal infection. If you think you have an infection, check with your doctor. If you want more information, please read in Chapter 10, <u>Vaginal Infections</u>.

- Intercourse may hurt for a few weeks or longer after you have a baby.
- Intercourse will hurt if your vagina is not wet enough. When you are sexually excited your vagina produces a fluid. This fluid is called lubrication because it lubricates, or wets, your vagina. It makes intercourse easier.

There are several reasons why you may not have enough lubrication. You may be rushing things. Most women do not get excited as quickly as men do. Many men are ready for intercourse before women are lubricated enough. Or, if you are going through menopause, or if you are past menopause, your body may not be producing enough lubrication.

If you want to have intercourse but you don't have enough lubrication, here are some things you can try:

- More Kissing and Touching.
  Kissing and touching are often called "foreplay". The word foreplay sounds as if kissing and touching are not as important as intercourse. However, for many women, kissing and touching are much more exciting than intercourse. Many women prefer them.

If you want to have intercourse, kissing and touching may make your vagina lubricated. Then intercourse should be painless. Tell or show your sexual partner what you want, and what you like.

- **Lubricating Jelly.**
Use a "washable lubricating jelly", such as K-Y jelly. You can buy lubricating jellies in a drugstore without a prescription.

Don't use petroleum jelly (Vaseline).

- It does not dissolve in water, and it cannot be washed away. It can trap bacteria in your vagina, and this can cause infections.

- Petroleum jelly can weaken condoms and diaphragms. If they have holes in them, condoms and diaphragms are not safe birth control.

- **Estrogen Cream during Menopause.**
If your vagina becomes drier during menopause, a lubricating jelly may help. If it doesn't help enough, estrogen creams can be very helpful. However, there are some dangers in using estrogen. (If you want more information about estrogen creams, please read p. 392 in Chapter 13, <u>Menopause</u>.)

Making love.

Making love means everything that people do when they have sex. When you make love, you may like kissing and touching and talking. You may also like intercourse, or oral sex or anal sex.

- **Sexual Intercourse.** Sexual intercourse is when the penis is in the vagina. It is usually just called intercourse.

- **Oral Sex.** Oral sex is touching your partner's sexual parts with your lips and tongue. Oral sex can be done by women or by men. It can be done to women or to men. Oral sex is normal, and it is very common. Both heterosexuals and homosexuals enjoy oral sex.

- **Anal Sex.** Anal sex means that the penis is in the anus, or near the anus. The area around your anus can be very sensitive, and some women like to be touched there. However, some women don't like anal intercourse, because it can hurt.
  Anal intercourse can lead to vaginal infections. This can happen if you have vaginal intercourse right after anal intercourse. Anal intercourse can also cause tears or rips in your anus. Always use condoms and a lubricant during anal intercourse. Remove the condom before you have vaginal intercourse.

You can make love whatever way you like, as long as you and your partner both want to do it.

Orgasms.

- When you are making love, sexual tension builds up. An orgasm is the very pleasant release of sexual tension. It is often called "coming", or a climax.

- Orgasms don't have to happen at the same time for both people. They seldom do. You may never have an orgasm at the same time as your partner, and that's OK.

- You don't have to have an orgasm every time you make love. Many people think that they have failed if they haven't had one. Love-making does not have to end with an orgasm for either person. Orgasms can be fun, but they are not necessary. Nothing is necessary besides caring about the other person.

- There is no right or wrong way to have an orgasm. You can have a orgasm from masturbation, from touching, from oral sex, or from vaginal intercourse. Experiment to see what works best for you. Many women have trouble having orgasms during intercourse. Masturbation, touching and oral sex work much better for them.

- Women can have several orgasms in a row. These are called "multiple orgasms". However, men need to wait a while after one orgasm before they can have another one.
- If you don't have orgasms easily, it doesn't mean that you are "frigid". Nobody is "frigid". Many women cannot have orgasms from intercourse alone.

There are many reasons why women don't have orgasms easily. You may be nervous, or your partner may not know what to do. Or, you and your partner may not be getting along. If the conditions are right, you can learn to have orgasms if you want to.

Some men call women "frigid" when they don't want to have sex with them. This is a way of forcing women to have sex. Don't ever let someone pressure you into having sex. It's always your choice.

Masturbation.

- Masturbation is rubbing or touching your own sexual parts for pleasure, or to produce an orgasm.
- Masturbation is OK for married people or single people.
- Both women and men masturbate.
- Both old people and young people masturbate.

- If a woman doesn't have orgasms easily, then masturbation can help her to learn how.
- Many people masturbate as part of love-making. Many do it sometimes instead of intercourse.
- Masturbation will not make you get sick or make you go crazy. It will not cause any harm at all.

Pregnancy.

- You can get pregnant even if you have sex only once.
- You can get pregnant without actually having intercourse. You can get pregnant without actually having a penis in your vagina. If even a little semen is released near your vagina, some of the sperm can get into your vagina. If even one sperm reaches an egg, you can get pregnant.
- Swallowing semen cannot cause pregnancy.
- Because sex can cause pregnancy, both you and your partner must think about birth control. (If you want more information about birth control, please read Chapter 9, Birth Control.)
- Many people think pregnant women should not have intercourse. This is not true. Intercourse is harmless during a normal pregnancy. Sex will not hurt or "mark" your baby.

However, if you have certain problems with your pregnancy, intercourse or orgasms can sometimes be harmful. Check with your doctor if you are not sure what you can do.

- Some women are not interested in sex when they are pregnant. This may be because sex is not comfortable. If you are interested in sex, but it is uncomfortable, try some different positions. You could try having intercourse on your sides, either facing each other or with the man behind you. If this doesn't help, check with your doctor.

- Before labour, or during labour, your waters will break. The "waters" is the bag of water the baby is floating in inside your uterus. After the waters break, your uterus is no longer sealed off. It is a little opened. You must not have intercourse after your waters have broken, because intercourse can cause an infection in your uterus.

Aging.

- Menopause does not mean the end of your sex life. Menopause does not mean that you will stop wanting or enjoying sex. (Remember, you can still get pregnant while you are going through menopause. You need at least a whole year without periods before you can stop using birth control.)

- If you choose to, you can have an active sex life until you die. Some older people continue to enjoy sex until their death. Some older people do not. This is either because they don't have partners, or because they are not interested. There is no physical reason why old people cannot enjoy sex.
- If getting older has caused a physical problem which makes sex difficult, talk with your doctor or with a sex therapist. Many of these problems can be overcome.

Men.

- When a man has an orgasm, he also "ejaculates". This means that fluid called semen comes out of his penis. This semen contains sperm.
- A hard penis is called an "erection". An erection does not mean that the man must have an orgasm. An erection does not mean he must ejaculate. He will not be harmed in any way if he doesn't ejaculate. He can always have another erection later. Don't let a man pressure you by saying that he must have sex or else something bad will happen to him. It won't.
- If a man cannot get an erection, it is not your fault. It is no one's fault. It happens to all men sometimes.

- The size of a penis has nothing to do with how much sex drive he has, or how good a lover he is.
- The penis and testicles are not the only sensitive places on a man's body. His ears, mouth, nipples, and buttocks are also sexually sensitive.

Fantasies.

- Most women have sexual fantasies at one time or another.
- Having fantasies does not mean that you are going to do them, or even that you want to do them.
- Most fantasies are harmless. However, fantasies can be a problem if you act them out in the real world.
- Remember: you don't have to act out your partner's fantasies if you don't want to.

Sexual assault.

- Sexual assault means forcing someone to have sex. It also means threatening to hurt someone if they won't have sex. Most people call sexual assault "rape". Rape is when a penis is forced into the vagina or the anus or the mouth.

- Incest is another kind of sexual assault. Incest is sexual abuse of children by someone in the family. Incest is much more common than we realize. One out of every three girls is assaulted while they are children. Also, one out of every five boys is assaulted.
- Sexual assault is very common. At least 1 in every 4 women in Canada is sexually assaulted during her lifetime. On average, one woman is raped in Canada every 17 minutes. This does <u>not</u> include being hassled by men on the street, or at your job, or other kinds of sexual harassment.
- Sexual assault is a violent crime. Rape is not sex; rape is violence. If someone - even your husband - forces you to have sex, this is rape.
- If you have been sexually assaulted, you can get help from a Rape Crisis Centre or a Sexual Assault Crisis Centre in your area. Their phone number is often in the front of the phone book. The police may also have their number.

You can call a Crisis Centre right after your attack. The workers at the Centre will give you support. They will also help you decide what to do next. You can also call a Centre to talk about an attack that happened a long time ago. Some Centres have support groups for women who were assaulted when they were children.

Sexually Transmitted Diseases.

The biggest worry people used to have about sex was pregnancy. Now there is another worry - disease. We cannot talk about sex without also talking about Sexually Transmitted Diseases, or STDs.

Sexually Transmitted Diseases are diseases which you get from sexual contact. They used to be called VD. Now they are called STDs. AIDS, chlamydia, gonorrhea, and herpes are all STDs.

Anyone who has sex can get an STD. When you have sex with someone, you could get the germs which they have. Some of these germs may cause STDs.

Think of it this way. If your partner has one other partner, then he may be carrying germs from this other person. Then, during sex, you can get the germs of two people, not one. And, if he or she had sex with others, then you could get these other people's germs too. And, if the other partner has had sex with others, you could get those other peoples' germs too. And so on and so on. Before you know it, even if you have only slept with one person, you could have come in contact with the germs of many, many other people. Not all these germs will cause an STD. However, some could.

So, the more people you sleep with, the greater your chances are of getting an STD.

You can't tell who will and who won't be carrying an STD. People can carry STD germs without being sick themselves. For example, a man can carry the chlamydia bacteria without having any symptoms. However, you could catch chlamydia from him and then develop a serious infection. This is why it is so important to know how to protect yourself. This is why using condoms is so important.

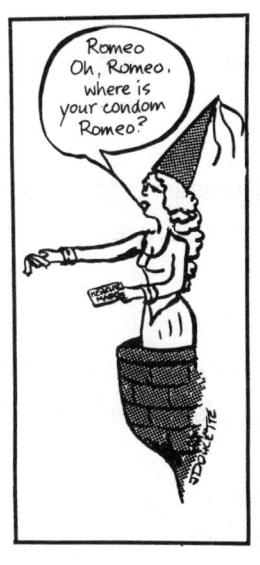

© J. Doucette, 1987

On the following pages there is information on each of these diseases. If you want more information, you could ask your doctor or your public health nurse. You could also call an STD or VD hotline. Most cities now have this kind of hotline.

AIDS.

"What is AIDS?"

AIDS is a disease caused by a virus. This virus attacks your body's immune system. Your immune system is very important because it fights diseases. A person with AIDS has a hard time fighting off diseases. They become sick very easily. They often get pneumonia or cancer, and usually they die of one of these diseases.

AIDS is very dangerous. There is no cure for AIDS, and there is no vaccine to protect you from getting it.

"How do I get AIDS?"

When a person is infected with AIDS, the AIDS virus is in their blood and in their semen. It is also found in smaller amounts in their vaginal fluid, tears, saliva and breast milk.

AIDS is spread when the virus from an infected person gets into another person's blood. This usually happens in one of these ways:

1. Unsafe Sex. AIDS is usually spread by having unsafe sex with an infected person. This is the most common way that AIDS is spread for both men and women.

2. Drug Needles. AIDS is also spread by using the needles and syringes of infected people. These are called I.V. drugs because they are injected into the veins. This is often called shooting up.

3. Pregnancy. AIDS can be spread from an infected pregnant mother to her baby.

4. Blood Transfusions. AIDS can be spread by infected blood during a blood transfusion. However, all blood in Canada is now tested for AIDS. Therefore, now there is very little danger of getting AIDS in a transfusion.

AIDS cannot be caught in everyday situations. It is not spread through air, water, food, or ordinary body contact. You cannot get AIDS by holding hands or hugging. You can't get AIDS by taking care of an infected person. You can't get AIDS from toilet seats or swimming pools. You can't get AIDS while giving blood.

After a person is infected with the AIDS virus, they do not get sick right away. Sometimes they have the virus in their body for several years without knowing it. This is very dangerous because these infected people can give the virus to others during this time. Although they may not feel sick, they can give AIDS to other people.

"How can I avoid getting AIDS?"
Anyone can get AIDS, whether you are heterosexual or homosexual. It all depends on what you do. If you take risks, you can get AIDS.

If you want to avoid AIDS, you have a couple of choices to make. To be completely safe, don't have sex at all. If you don't want to do this, then only have sex with one safe person. Make sure this person does not have AIDS now, and make sure that they won't be able to catch it and pass it on to you. That is, make sure that they do not have <u>any other</u> sexual partners — men or women. Also, make sure that they do not shoot up drugs. If you are not sure about your partner or partners, then you need to know about "Safer Sex".

Safer Sex.

Safer Sex means that you don't do anything which would let the AIDS virus get into your body. This means that you must not come in contact with your partner's semen or blood. If your partner has AIDS, you could become infected. If you have a tiny cut in your vagina, or your mouth or your anus, then the virus could get from their semen or blood into your blood.

If you follow the rules of "Safer Sex", you will prevent the AIDS virus from getting into your body.

Rules for Safer Sex.

Safer Sex means using condoms. Some people don't like condoms. Even if you or your partner don't like them, remember this: they could save your lives. If your partner doesn't want to use a condom, you may have to insist. You could tell him, "No condom, no sex". When you ask a man to use a condom, you are not accusing him of anything. What you are doing is protecting your health, and maybe his too. If you are close enough to have sex with someone, then you should be close enough to talk about Safer Sex.

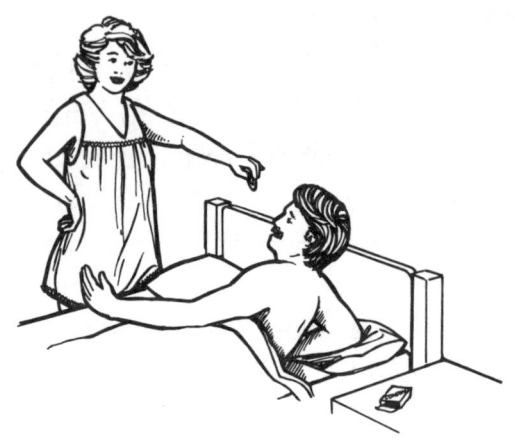

1. Don't have sex with anyone unless you are sure they don't have AIDS. The more partners, the more risks. Unless you are <u>sure</u> about your partner, use a condom every time you have sex.

2. For extra protection, either use condoms which have a spermicidal lubricant, or use a spermicidal birth control foam with the condom. Spermicides kill the AIDS virus. They may also kill the germs which cause other STDs — herpes, chlamydia and gonorrhea. (If you want to know more about using spermicidal foam, please read p. 278, in Chapter 9 <u>Birth Control</u>.)

3. Don't have sex with people who use needle drugs such as heroin and speed.

4. Don't shoot up drugs yourself. These drugs are dangerous, and because of AIDS, they are even more dangerous. If you use them, don't share your needles and syringes with anyone else.

Using condoms the right way.

Many people make mistakes when they use condoms. Here are some rules to remember:

- Have condoms ready to use for every time you have sex.
- Use a condom for vaginal, oral and anal intercourse.
- Use good, latex condoms. Do not use natural condoms. They can let the AIDS virus pass through them.
- Open the package carefully so you don't tear the condom.
- Leave a space at the end to hold the semen. Pinch the space to get the air out.
- Put the condom on as soon as his penis is erect. Do not wait until just before intercourse.
- Afterwards, the man should pull out right away. He should hold onto the condom at the base of his penis to prevent any semen from spilling out.
- Only use a water-soluble lubricant. Never use Vaseline. Vaseline can weaken the latex in condoms.
- Never use the same condom more than once.

Safer Sex is very important; it can keep you healthy. Even though condoms do break once in a while, Safer Sex is much safer than sex without any protection.

Remember, it is very risky to have lots of partners, and it is risky to have a partner who has other partners. If you want to avoid AIDS, don't use I.V. drugs, and use a condom every time you have sex.

If you or your partner(s) have used I.V. drugs, OR if your partner is bisexual, OR if you have had lots of partners you should likely be tested for AIDS. If you think you or your partner may have AIDS don't wait for symptoms. Go and get tested. The earlier you find out, the better your chances are. And, the earlier you find out, the less chance you have of spreading AIDS to someone else.

AIDS is a new disease. New information about AIDS is discovered all the time. If you want more information about AIDS, you could ask your public health nurse or your doctor. You could also contact an AIDS organization in your area. Some provinces have AIDS information hotlines. These hotlines are run by the Ministry or Department of Health. You can find these numbers in the Blue Pages of your phone book. Look under Health-Ministry or Health-Department in the Provincial Government section.

Chlamydia. (This is pronounced kluh-MID-ee-ah.)

"What is chlamydia?"

Chlamydia is now a very common STD. It is spread by sexual intercourse.

A chlamydia infection is very serious because it can cause Pelvic Inflammatory Disease, or, P.I.D.. P.I.D. is a serious infection in your uterus which can make you unable to get pregnant. (If you want more information on P.I.D., please read p. 263 in this chapter.)

"How will I know if I have chlamydia?"

- You may have a vaginal discharge. Your discharge may be heavy or light. It may be creamy or yellow.
- You may have unusual bleeding, or deep pain after intercourse.
- You may also have pain when you pass urine (pee). If it hurts to pee, then the infection has spread to your bladder. This is called "cystitis".

However, you may have chlamydia without any of these signs. You may not know you have chlamydia until it has spread to your uterus. A man with chlamydia will often have burning or pain when he pees.

"How do I get rid of chlamydia?"

If you have any signs of a chlamydia infection, go to your doctor. Your doctor will give you either tetracycline or erythromycin. Make sure that you finish the whole prescription.

Your sexual partner must be treated also. In the meantime, and if sex is not painful, use condoms until you are both cured. When your prescription is finished, go back to your doctor. You need to have another test to see if you are cured.

Chlamydia is a serious infection. If you have a new male partner, and you get a vaginal infection or pain in your abdomen, be sure to ask your doctor to test you for chlamydia. If your partner has a bladder infection, ask your doctor to test you for chlamydia. Better to be safe than sorry.

"How can I avoid getting chlamydia?"

- The more partners, the more risk.
- Use condoms and contraceptive foam.
- Don't have sex with a man who has discharge from his penis, or pain when he pees.
- If you have several sexual partners, ask your doctor to do a culture for chlamydia at least once a year.
- If you want to know more about how to avoid STDs, please read p. 268 in this chapter.

Gonorrhea.

"What is gonorrhea?"

Gonorrhea is a common, serious STD. It is sometimes called "clap". Gonorrhea is spread by intercourse. It can be spread by vaginal or anal intercourse, or during oral sex.

If gonorrhea is not treated, it can cause Pelvic Inflammatory Disease, P.I.D.. (If you want more information on P.I.D., please read p. 263 in this chapter.)

"How will I know if I have gonorrhea?"

- Some women with gonorrhea have a thick vaginal discharge.
- However, most women do not know anything is wrong until the infection is serious. By then the infection is in their uterus and tubes. Then they have severe pain in their lower abdomen. They may also have pain when they pee (pass urine).
- Men with gonorrhea usually have a discharge from their penis, and pain when they pee (pass urine).

"How do I get rid of gonorrhea?"

If you have gonorrhea, you will likely get either an injection of penicillin or penicillin tablets. Sometimes you may get tetracycline instead. Finish your whole prescription, and use condoms until you are sure your infection is gone.

When your prescription is finished, go back to your doctor. Have another test to see if you are cured. All of your partners must also be treated.

"How can I avoid getting gonorrhea?"

• The more partners, the more risk.

• Use condoms and contraceptive foam.

• Don't have sex with a man who has discharge from his penis, or pain when he pees.

• If you have several sexual partners, ask your doctor to do a culture for gonorrhea at least once a year.

• If you want to know more about how to avoid STDs, please read p. 268 in this chapter.

Herpes.

"What is herpes?"

Herpes is caused by a virus. This virus is similar to the virus which causes cold sores. Herpes is spread by sexual contact.

Herpes is a problem for these four reasons:

1. Herpes causes blisters which hurt a lot.

2. Women with herpes may be more likely to get cancer of the cervix. Women with herpes should have a Pap test every 6 months. (If you want more information on Pap Tests, please read Chapter 11, <u>Pap Tests</u>.)

3. Herpes can be dangerous for pregnant women. If you catch herpes during your pregnancy, your baby may also get herpes. A herpes infection can be very harmful to your baby.

If you already have herpes before you get pregnant, there is less risk. However, there is some risk for your baby if you have a herpes blister at delivery time.

Be sure to tell your doctor if you have or have had herpes.

4. You can easily spread herpes to your sexual partners.

"How will I know if I have it?"
The first time you have herpes, you will likely be quite sick. You may have a fever and pain around your lower abdomen and thighs. Small red bumps will appear on or near your vagina. Then these bumps will become very painful, open blisters. It can become very painful to pee (pass urine). The blisters heal in about two weeks. You may not feel well until the blisters are all gone.

Herpes is usually easy to diagnose. Your doctor should take a swab from a sore and send it to the laboratory to be sure.

After the blisters have gone, the virus does not go away. It stays in your body forever. From time to time it can produce new sores again. In this way it is similar to cold sores.

Some people have only one outbreak of herpes. However, most people have other attacks. These second attacks are less serious. If you have a second attack, you will have fewer blisters and they will hurt less. Usually you will not have a fever, and you will not feel very sick. As time goes by, you will likely have fewer outbreaks.

No one is sure what brings on these other attacks of herpes. Sometimes they happen when you are under stress, or after you are in the sun too much. Sometimes they happen before your menstrual period, and sometimes if you are sick or run down.

You must not have any sexual contact when your blisters are full of fluid. If you do, you can easily spread herpes. You can also keep spreading it until your sores have healed over. You may even be able to spread it when you are getting a sore, but this is not known. You can have sex again when your sores are healed.

"How do I get rid of herpes?"
- There is no cure for herpes. You have the virus in your body for life.
- While you are waiting for your blisters to heal, keep the area warm and dry so that the blisters do not get infected. Warm baths will help ease the pain. Some women have so much pain that they have to pee in a tub of warm water. This prevents the urine from touching their open sores. Your doctor can also give you something for the pain.

- You may feel embarrassed to tell your new partners that you have herpes. Remember: many people either have it or have been in contact with it. Try to remember that you will be doing everyone a favour by telling the truth. Be responsible.

"How can I avoid getting herpes?"
- The more partners, the more risk.
- Condoms and contraceptive foam may help to keep it from spreading. However, they are no guarantee.
- Don't have sex if you or your partner has open blisters.
- If you want to know more about how to avoid STDs, please read p. 268 in this chapter.

Pelvic Inflammatory Disease (P.I.D.)

If you have chlamydia or gonorrhea, and you don't get it treated, you can become very sick. The infection can move up into your uterus and tubes. This drawing shows how your vagina leads up to your uterus. This is where the infection can travel to.

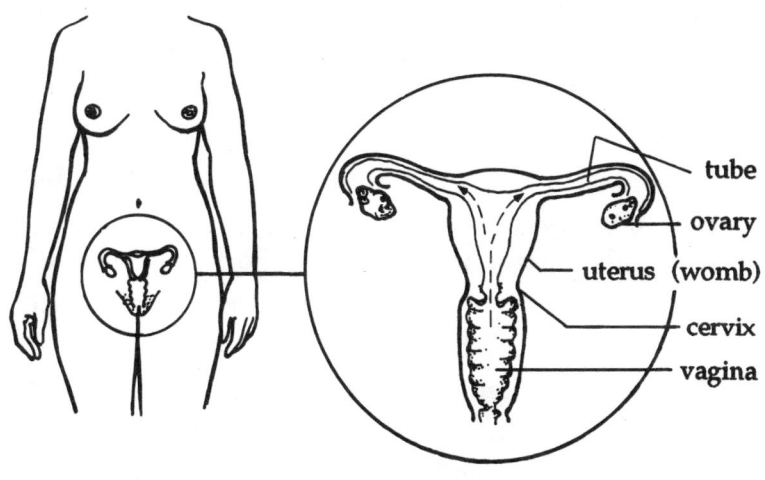

tube
ovary
uterus (womb)
cervix
vagina

This kind of infection is called Pelvic Inflammatory Disease, or P.I.D. P.I.D. is very common. It is also very serious.

P.I.D. must be treated with antibiotics. If it is not treated early, it can cause these very serious problems:

- **P.I.D. can make you very sick.**
  You may need to go into a hospital to get special antibiotics. You might even need to have an operation to drain the abscesses. Before antibiotics, women used to die of P.I.D..

- **P.I.D. can make it impossible for you to get pregnant.**
  Your tubes can become permanently blocked because of the scar tissue from the infection. If your tubes are blocked, the egg and the sperm cannot reach each other to start a pregnancy.

- **P.I.D. can make you more likely to have tubal pregnancies.**
  In a tubal pregnancy, the egg does not start to grow in your uterus (or womb) where it should. Instead, it starts to grow in one of your tubes. This is a problem because the egg cannot grow to full size in a tube. If you have a tubal pregnancy, you will need to have an emergency operation to remove it. If you didn't have this operation, the tube would burst, and you could die. Tubal pregnancies are also called "ectopic" pregnancies.

- **P.I.D. can cause severe, long-lasting pain in your lower abdomen.**

"How will I know if I have P.I.D.?"

P.I.D. is very dangerous because you can have it without knowing it. Many women have it for a long time before they realize it. By then, they may have a very serious infection. Some women don't find out they have had P.I.D. until they find out that they can't get pregnant.

Here are some of the signs of P.I.D. which you should look out for:

- pain in your lower abdomen
- unusual discharge from your vagina
- fever or chills
- a feeling of being very sick, like the flu
- painful sex
- bleeding after sex
- pain in your back or legs
- pain when you pee
- bleeding from your vagina in between periods.

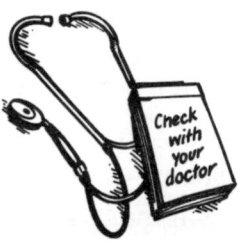

If you have one or more of these symptoms, you may have P.I.D.. The only way to be sure is to have a doctor examine you. The examination plus some lab tests will tell for sure if you have P.I.D..

"Who is likely to get P.I.D.?"

Some women have a greater chance of getting P.I.D.. If you are one of these women, know the signs, and get a check-up to be sure.

1. Women who have several sexual partners are more likely to get P.I.D..

Women with many partners are more likely to get P.I.D. because they are more likely to get a Sexually Transmitted Disease (STD) from their partners. STDs can lead to P.I.D.. The more partners you or your partner have, the greater your risk of getting P.I.D.. If you have P.I.D. you should tell all your sexual partners. Tell them the kind of the infection which caused your P.I.D.. They should also be treated so that the infection is not passed back and forth.

2. Women who have an IUD (a coil) are more likely to get P.I.D..

The string of the IUD leads from your uterus into your vagina. This string lets bacteria travel from your vagina up into your uterus.

3. Women who have had P.I.D. before are more likely to get P.I.D. again.

These women often have a harder time getting rid of it the second time.

4. **Women who douche often are more likely to get P.I.D..**
Douching can force bacteria up into your uterus. The best advice is "Don't douche". If you want to douche sometimes, only use a very low pressure douche.

5. **Women who have had many D. and C.s or several abortions are more likely to get P.I.D..**
Women can sometimes get infections during these operations.

If you think you may have P.I.D., see your doctor now. If you get treated quickly, you have a much better chance of being cured. If you get treated quickly, you have a much better chance of avoiding a long-lasting problem.

If you have P.I.D., you may not be sick enough to be in hospital. Even if you don't feel really sick, put yourself to bed and stay there. This means complete bed rest until you are cured. If you have an IUD, have it removed.

"How can I avoid getting P.I.D.?"
P.I.D. is caused by an STD. To avoid getting P.I.D. you have to avoid getting an STD.

How to avoid STDs:

- Know your sexual partners.
- Use condoms and contraceptive foam, even if you have another method of birth control. Condoms prevent infected semen from getting into your vagina. The chemicals in the foam also kill some germs. Some condoms are lubricated with spermicidal lubricant. These chemicals also kill the germs which cause P.I.D.
- Don't have sex with anyone if they have any signs of infection. It's hard to know for sure if someone has an infection because you can't always see signs of an STD. However, look for a discharge or any unusual sores. Ask your partner if she or he has pain when they pee (pass urine). Ask a woman partner if she has an unusual discharge. If you want to be sure, you may want your partner to have a test first.
- Put a limit on the number of people you have sex with. The more partners, the more likely you will get an STD.
- If you have several partners, and if you want to get pregnant in the future, don't use an IUD. If you have an IUD, you increase your chances of getting P.I.D.

- If you have more than one partner, or if your partner has other partners, have STD tests at least once a year. If you have many partners, get checked more than once a year.
- If you find out you have an STD, let all your sexual partners know. They should also be treated.
- You can get gonorrhea or chlamydia again. If you have had them once, you can get them again.
- Don't be shy. Take care of your health by talking about these things with the people you have sex with.

Remember, love and sex do not always go together.
- Someone may want to have sex with you, but they may not love you or even care about you at all.
- You may love someone and not want to have sex with them.
- You may want a sexual relationship with someone that you don't love.
- You may love someone a lot, and you may want to make love with them.

Make sure that you know what you are doing, and make your choices carefully.

Remember: you can decide what you do about sex. It is your choice. You have the right to choose, and the right to be respected for your choice.

Birth Control

9

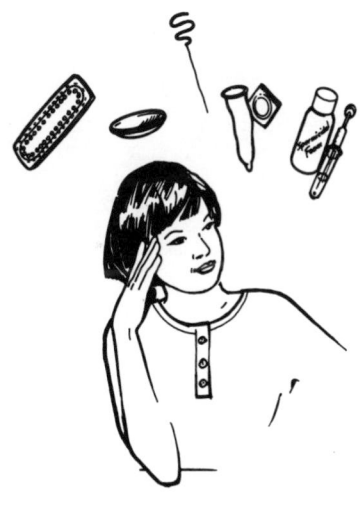

BIRTH CONTROL

Nowadays there are many different birth control methods to choose from. These methods will prevent most pregnancies. However, no method is 100% safe. The more you know about how to use your method, the better it will work for you.

If you want to make your method work well for you, you need to understand how a pregnancy can happen.

How pregnancy happens.

Unless you are already pregnant, every month your body gets ready to get pregnant.

First the lining of your uterus (or womb) starts to thicken. Then an egg starts to grow in one ovary. One or two weeks later, the tiny egg is released. The time when the egg is released is called "ovulation".

After the egg is released, it travels down a tube towards your uterus. This is the time when you can get pregnant. It is called your "fertile" time. This is usually about two weeks <u>before</u> your next period.

You may also notice a change in your vaginal discharge at this time. At ovulation, this discharge is clear and slippery, and it looks like raw egg white. Because it is produced when you are "fertile", it is called "fertile mucus". This mucus helps the sperm travel up into your uterus.

When you have intercourse, millions of sperm are released in your vagina. This happens unless your partner has had a vasectomy, or unless he is using a condom. These sperm then travel up into your uterus and tubes. If a sperm joins with the egg, then the egg is called "a fertilized egg". This is the beginning of a pregnancy.

The fertilized egg then moves down the tube to your uterus. Then it attaches itself to the inside of the uterus. The fertilized egg is now called an "embryo". It will continue to grow there for nine months until it is a baby, and it is ready to be born.

If the egg is not fertilized, the thick lining of your uterus is not needed. About two weeks later, your body gets rid of this lining. It comes out of your body though your vagina. This is called "having your menstrual period", or "having your period", or "menstruating". The unused egg is also lost with your menstrual blood.

How birth control works.

Most birth control methods try to prevent the egg from ever meeting the sperm.

- **The Pill** prevents any eggs from being released.
- **The diaphragm** and **the condom and foam** are called "barrier methods". They put up a barrier which prevents sperm from getting into the uterus.
- **Tubal ligation** cuts the tubes which carry the eggs from the ovaries to the uterus. This prevents the eggs from reaching any sperm.
- **Vasectomy** cuts the tubes which carry sperm inside the man's body. This prevents any sperm from being released.
- **Natural Family Planning** prevents pregnancy by avoiding intercourse when an egg can be fertilized.
- **Withdrawal** prevents pregnancy by preventing most of the sperm from getting into the vagina.

The IUD does not prevent the egg and the sperm from meeting. It prevents the fertilized egg from starting to grow in the uterus.

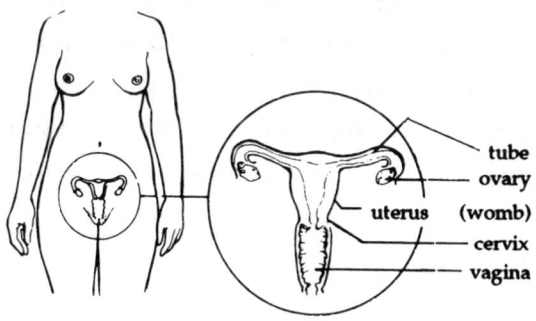

tube
ovary
uterus (womb)
cervix
vagina

How to choose the right method for you.

Choosing the best birth control method can be hard. There is no perfect method. Some methods work much better than others. Some methods are safer than others, and some are much easier to use than others.

Here are some questions which might help you decide on the best method for you:

- How often do I need birth control?
- Which method can I depend on the most?
- Which method is the safest for me?
- Which method has the least side effects?
- Which method is the easiest to use?
- Which method can I afford?

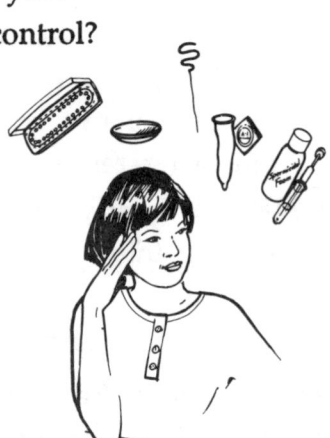

- Which method do I like and feel comfortable with?
- Which method will my partner like and feel comfortable with? (No method will work if you are too embarrassed to use it.)
- Is there any risk to my health if I get pregnant?
- What would I do if I got pregnant?

If you want more help in choosing, you could talk with a family planning worker, or a public health nurse, or a family doctor. You could also go to a women's health centre or clinic. Family Planning Clinics are usually run by a Health Unit. Find out all you can about each method. Then choose the one which suits you best.

If you have a regular sexual partner, take him along to the appointment. The more you both know about your method, the more you will both take responsibility for making it work. The more you both know about it, the better it will work for you.

Common birth control methods.

In this chapter you will find information about the most popular kinds of birth control. You can compare the methods based on how well they work, and how safe they are. You can also compare them based on how convenient they are, and how much they cost.

Remember, you don't have to have intercourse every time you make love. For example, you may decide not to have intercourse at all when you are most fertile. You can only get pregnant with vaginal intercourse. Kissing and touching and other kinds of love-making are good methods of birth control to use sometimes.

Condoms and Foam.

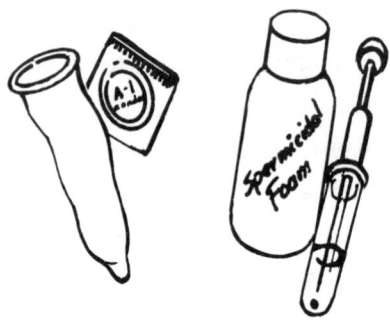

"What are condoms and foam?"
Condoms are coverings which fit over an erect penis. They are made of either latex (rubber) or animal tissue.

Foam is a soft cream which you place in your vagina before intercourse. It is called a "contraceptive" or "spermicidal" foam. It contains a chemical which kills the sperm.

Condoms and foam should be used together. **Together** they are almost as good at preventing pregnancy as the birth control pill.

Some condoms are lubricated with a spermicidal lubricant. The chemicals in the lubricant are useful because they kill both the sperm and the germs which cause sexually transmitted diseases.

"How do condoms and foam work?"
Condoms and foam are called a "barrier method" of birth control. The condom is a barrier which stops the sperm from getting into your vagina.

When the man ejaculates (or "comes"), semen comes out of his penis. This semen contains sperm. If the man is wearing a condom, the semen is caught inside the condom. This means that no sperm can get into your vagina. If the condom breaks, or if any of the semen leaks out of the condom, the sperm are killed by the foam.

"How well do condoms and foam work?"
Using condoms or foam by themselves are risky.
- When women use foam without condoms, about 20 out of every 100 women get pregnant.
- When women use condoms without foam, about 10 out of every 100 women get pregnant.

However, together they are very good birth control.
- When women use <u>both</u> condoms and foam, only about 4 out of every 100 women get pregnant. (If women use no birth control for a year, between 50 and 85 of them will get pregnant.)

"What is the right way to use condoms and foam?"
Using Foam:

- The foam must be inserted in your vagina <u>before</u> intercourse. It must be inserted no more than 30 minutes before the man ejaculates.
- Foam is not hard to use. Carefully read the directions on the container, and follow the directions exactly.
  - Shake the container 20 times to mix it well. Then fill the applicator with foam.
  - Insert the full applicator as far as possible into your vagina. Then pull it back about half an inch. Press the plunger. Foam will be released near the opening to your uterus. Then remove the applicator without pulling back on the plunger.
- If you make love a second time, you need to put in more foam, and you need a new condom.
- Some doctors advise women to use two applicators of foam during the first six months after they have a baby.
- Afterwards, the foam may drip out of your vagina. You may need to wear a panty liner to absorb it.
- Do not douche for at least eight hours afterwards. Douching can wash out the foam. (Douching is useless as a birth control method.)

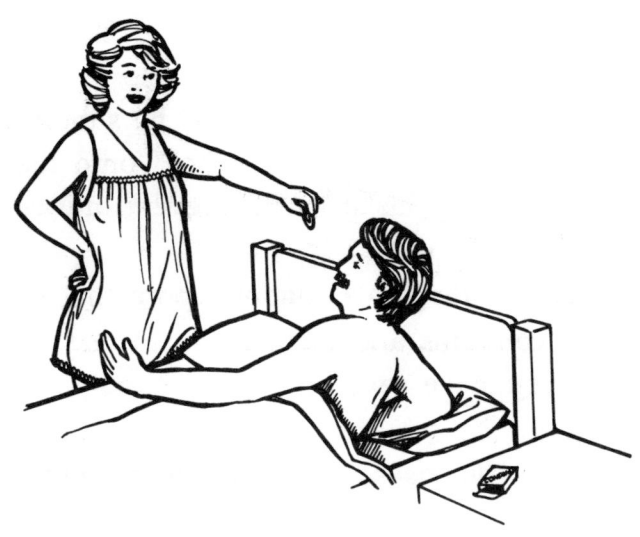

Using a condom:

• The man should put on a condom as soon as he has an erection. Do not wait until just before intercourse to put on the condom. The liquid which comes out of his penis before he ejaculates also contains sperm. You must not allow his penis to touch your vagina unless it is covered with a condom.

• Open the package carefully so you don't tear the condom. Unroll it carefully onto the penis. Leave a space at the end to hold the semen. Pinch the space to get the air out.

• If the condom is not lubricated, only use a water-soluble lubricant. Never use Vaseline. Vaseline can weaken the latex in condoms.

• If the condom tears, or if it comes off during intercourse, you must insert another applicator of foam right away.

- As soon as the man ejaculates, he should pull out of your vagina. He should hold onto the condom at the base of his penis to prevent any semen from spilling out.
- Never use the same condom more than once.
- Have condoms and foam ready to use for every time you have sex.

"What are the risks to my health if I use condoms and foam?"
- There are no health risks which we know about in using foam and condoms.
- However, some people are allergic to the chemicals in the foam and the spermicidal lubricant. They can irritate both your vagina and the man's penis.
- Some people are allergic to the latex in condoms. These people could use natural condoms instead. Natural condoms are made from animal tissue. However, natural condoms do not protect as well against AIDS.
- Besides preventing pregnancy, condoms and foam can help to protect your health. Condoms and foam can stop you from catching sexually transmitted diseases such as chlamydia, gonorrhea and AIDS. (If you want more information about sexually transmitted diseases, please read p. 246 in Chapter 8, Sex.)

"How convenient are condoms and foam?"
You need to have them ready every time you have
sex. This may take a little time to get used to. It
may also take time to get used to talking to your
partner about birth control. Remember, birth control
is something for both people to be concerned about.

"Where can I get condoms and foam?"
Buying Condoms:
- You do not need a prescription for condoms. You
  can buy condoms at a drug store, or from a
  vending machine. You can also get them free at
  some birth control clinics.

Buying Foam:
- You can also buy foam without a prescription.
  You can buy foam in a drug store or at a birth
  control clinic. Drug stores also sell creams and
  jellies which kill sperm. However, foam kills
  sperm best.
- Make sure that you buy foam which is called
  "contraceptive" or "spermicidal" foam. Make sure
  that you are not buying a "feminine hygiene"
  douche or perfume. These are useless for birth
  control. (They are just plain useless.) In some
  drug stores contraceptive foams are kept near the
  feminine hygiene products. In others stores, they
  are near the condoms.

- When you buy your first package of foam, make sure it contains an applicator.
- When you buy foam, check the expiry date. It tells you when it is no longer good.
- It is a good idea to have an extra can of foam on hand. There is no way to know when your container is nearly empty.

"How much do condoms and foam cost?"
Condoms cost from 40¢ to 90¢ each, depending on the kind. Plain condoms are the cheapest. Natural condoms, lubricated condoms, and condoms with spermicidal lubricant cost more. All of them are tested and safe to use for birth control. You will save money if you buy the large boxes of condoms.

A small can of foam costs about $18.50. It contains enough foam for 10 to 15 applications. Foam is not cheap. But, if you use it with condoms, it is very good birth control. Remember, you and your partner should share the cost of birth control.

"Can I still get pregnant in the future if I use condoms and foam?"
If you use foam and condoms, you will still be able to get pregnant in the future.

The Birth Control Pill.

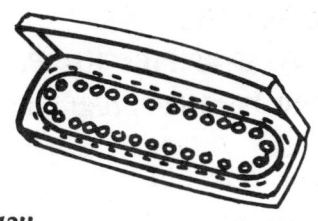

"What is the Pill?"

Birth control pills contain two hormones: estrogen and progesterone. These are similar to the hormones which are made naturally in your body. These hormones control your menstrual periods.

Birth control pills are also called "oral contraceptives".

"How does the Pill work?"

The Pill works by preventing your ovaries from releasing an egg every month. If no eggs are released, then you cannot get pregnant.

"How well does the Pill work?"

The Pill is one of the most reliable kinds of birth control. Only about 2 out of every 100 women get pregnant while they are taking the Pill. Most of these women get pregnant because of a mistake, such as forgetting to take a pill.

"What is the right way to use the Pill?"

Rules for taking the Pill.

It is very important to take the Pill correctly. If you do not, you may become pregnant.

1. You must take one pill every day, whether you are having sex or not. If you take one pill every day at the same time, you will keep a steady amount of hormones in your body. This will prevent any eggs from being released from your ovaries.

Choose a regular time to take your pill, and make it a habit. Some women take their pills first thing every morning. If the Pill upsets their stomach, some take it before bed. Choose a time that you will be able to remember and stick to it.

2. Start your package of pills on the exact day your doctor told you to. If you are not sure, ask until you are. Get your instructions in writing to help you remember.

3. Take one pill a day until the package is finished.

4. If you miss your period, and if you are sure that you have not missed any pills, don't worry. Start your next package of pills on schedule. Chances are very low that you are pregnant. You could have a pregnancy test if you are worried.

5. If you want to stop taking the Pill, check with your doctor, or check with your birth control counsellor.

- If you don't want to get pregnant, they will tell you when to stop taking the Pill.
- If you want to get pregnant, they may tell you to use another birth control method until you have had one or two periods. Then you can start trying to get pregnant.

6. During the first month of taking the Pill, you might still get pregnant. Many doctors suggest that you also use another kind of birth control, such as foam and condoms, during the first month. With the Pill plus an extra method you have almost no chance of getting pregnant.

Missing a Pill.

- If you miss one pill, take it as soon as you remember. Then take the next pill at your regular time. Use another method of birth control, such as condoms and foam, until your next period.
- If you miss two pills, take them as soon as you remember. Then take two the next day. Also use another method of birth control until your next period.

- If you miss more than two pills, call your doctor and follow his or her advice.
- If you vomit, you might throw up the Pill. If you have diarrhea, the Pill might not be absorbed into your body. If you are vomiting or have diarrhea, call your doctor. Ask her or him whether you should take extra pills. Ask if you should also use another kind of birth control.
- If you miss one or more pills and don't get your period, call your doctor. You may be pregnant, so you must not take any more pills. The hormones in the pills could hurt the embryo.

If you break up with your boyfriend or partner, don't go off the Pill right away. Lots of women get pregnant when they "make up" with their boyfriends. Stay on the Pill until you are sure that you are not going to need it. Stay on the Pill until you are sure that you are not going to have any sexual partners for a long time.

"How convenient is the Pill?"
The Pill is very easy to use. Always take it every day at the same time of day.

"What are the risks to my health if I use the Pill?"
There are some health risks in taking the Pill. There are also health risks in getting pregnant. These risks are greater for some women than for others.

Think carefully before you decide to take the Pill. Compare the risk of each birth control method with the risk of getting pregnant. This will help you find the best method for you.

If you want to take the Pill, first ask your doctor for a complete check-up. Your doctor should ask you about your medical history. Your doctor should also take your blood pressure and do a Pap test. All of this information will help you and your doctor decide if the Pill is safe for you.

The Pill is safer for some women than for others. This list may help you decide if the Pill is safe for you.

(1) You should not take the Pill if you have these health problems:
- high blood pressure
- cancer in your breast, uterus, or ovaries
- blood clots
- phlebitis, or poor circulation
- heart disease
- stroke
- liver disease
- unusual bleeding from your vagina

(2) You should think carefully about the risks of taking the Pill if you have these health problems:
- kidney disease
- fibroids in your uterus
- diabetes
- epilepsy
- asthma
- migraines
- severe depression
- very infrequent periods, (only 2 or 3 a year.)

If you are on the Pill and you have any of these problems, be sure to see your doctor for regular checkups.

(3) You should not take the Pill if you smoke.

If you smoke and take the Pill, you may have a dangerous combination. Smoking and the Pill both increase your chances of having a stroke, blood clots and a heart attack. Most women who have a heart attack while they are taking the Pill are smokers. The older you are, the greater the risk. If you are over 30, either stop smoking, or stop taking the Pill.

(4) You should not take the Pill if you are breast-feeding.

(5) You should stop taking the pill when you are 35.

(6) You should stop taking the Pill if you are going to have major surgery in the next four weeks.

Side Effects of the Pill

Side effects are extra ways that a drug affects you. These are different from the effects that the drug is supposed to have.

The Pill can affect many parts of your body. If you take the Pill, it is important to eat well. If you want to know more about special foods for women on the Pill, please read p. 33, in Chapter 1, Eating Well.

• **Harmful Side Effects of the Pill.**
The Pill can cause some harmful side effects. Some
of these are serious, but many of them are not.

- **Serious harmful side effects of the Pill.**
These side effects are serious, but
they are <u>not</u> very common:
- stroke
- high blood pressure
- blood clots
- depression
- jaundice

If the Pill is causing a serious side effect, you will
have some warning signs. If you have any of these
warning signs, **call your doctor right away:**

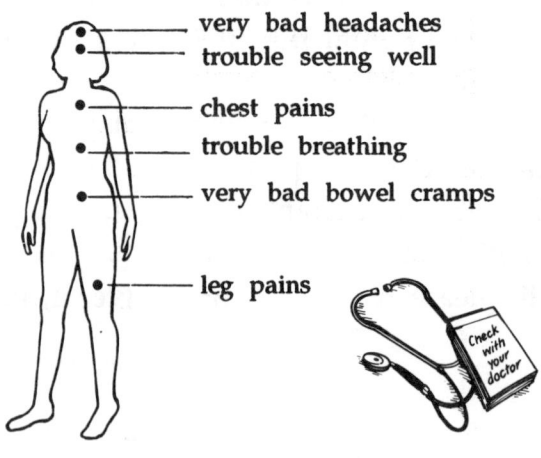

very bad headaches
trouble seeing well
chest pains
trouble breathing
very bad bowel cramps
leg pains

- Minor side effects of the Pill.

These minor side effects go away after two or three packages of pills:

- sore breasts
- tiredness
- nausea (sick stomach)
- weight gain
- bleeding (spotting) between periods
- bloating
- mild headaches
- acne
- yeast infections

• Helpful Side Effects of the Pill.

Besides being convenient birth control, the Pill can make some good changes in your health.

- If you take the Pill, you will have lighter periods. When you bleed less, you lose less iron. Then you won't get anemic as easily.
- If you take the Pill, you will probably have no menstrual cramps.
- If you take the Pill, you will have less chance of getting P.I.D., Pelvic Inflammatory Disease. (If you want to know more about P.I.D., please read p. 263, in Chapter 8, Sex.)
- If you take the Pill, you may have less chance of getting cysts or cancer in your ovaries.

- If you take the Pill, you may have less chance of getting some kinds of breast problems.
- If you take the Pill, you may have less chance of getting cancer in your uterus.

After looking at the pros and cons, many doctors and many women have decided this:

Low-dose pills are a good birth control method for healthy women under 35 who do not smoke.

If you take the Pill, ask for a low-dose kind. (Low-dose pills contain about 35 micrograms of estrogen.) And, while you are taking the Pill, have a complete medical check-up every year.

Remember, the Pill is a kind of medication. If you go to a doctor for another problem, tell the doctor that you are on the Pill.

"Can I still get pregnant in the future if I take the Pill?"

If you take the Pill, it will likely be easy for you to get pregnant in the future. If you want to get pregnant, your doctor will likely tell you to wait a few months. You may need to use another birth control method until you have had one or two periods. Then you can start trying to get pregnant.

"Where can I get the Pill?"

You need a prescription from a doctor to get the Pill. Never take your friend's pills.

"How much does the Pill cost?"

They cost from $13 to $16 per month. They are covered by some drug plans. Pills are much cheaper at birth control or family planning clinics.

The IUD.

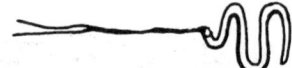

"What is an IUD?"
IUD stands for Intrauterine Device. An IUD is a device (or gadget) that is placed in your uterus (or womb). The IUD is just a small plastic coil with a string attached to it. Some IUDs are covered in thin copper wire. Some IUDs also contain a hormone called progesterone. An IUD is often called a "loop" or a "coil".

"How does an IUD work?"
No one is sure how an IUD works. It seems to prevent the fertilized egg from starting to grow in your uterus.

"How well does an IUD work?"
Only 3 or 4 women in every 100 will get pregnant with an IUD, as long as the IUD stays in.

"What is the right way to use an IUD?"
1. An IUD is inserted by a doctor. It is usually inserted during your period when your cervix is a little wider. (Your cervix is the opening to your uterus, or womb.) You may have cramps for a few hours after it is put in.

This drawing shows an IUD in place:

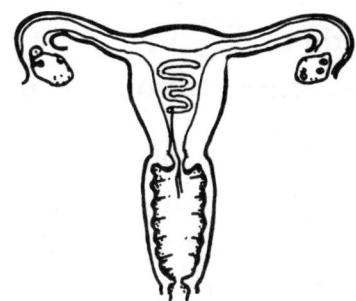

2. Before you leave the doctor's office, be sure that you know how to check for the IUD string. This is very important. It is the only way for you to know if the IUD is still in place.

Usually IUDs stay in place. However, sometimes they come back down through the cervix.
- You should be able to feel the string at the back of your vagina. It should feel the same as it did in the doctor's office.
- If you cannot find the string, the IUD may not be in place.
- If you can feel the plastic coil, or if the string is much longer, your IUD is not in place.
- If you have bleeding or pain during intercourse, your IUD may not be in place.
- If you have severe cramping, your IUD may not be in place.

If your IUD is not in place, you can get pregnant. If you think your IUD is out of place:
- Call your doctor right away.
- If you need birth control, use another method.

3. IUDs are more often pushed out during the first three months after they are put in. Because of this, many women use another method of birth control for the first three months. Many women use foam and condoms during this time.

4. For extra protection, some women with an IUD use foam and condoms every month at the time when they are fertile.

5. You can become pregnant with your IUD still in place, but this is not common. If you think you may be pregnant, go to your doctor at once. If you are pregnant, your doctor will likely want to remove the IUD. If it is not removed, you have a higher chance of getting an infection. This infection can cause a miscarriage.

6. An IUD must be removed by a doctor. Never try to remove it yourself.

7. You should not be able to feel your IUD when it is in place. Your sexual partner should also not be able to feel your IUD when it is in place. It will not be in the way when you are using tampons.

"What are the risks to my health if I use an IUD?"
If you have an IUD, you have a bigger risk of getting Pelvic Inflammatory Disease. IUDs can also cause heavier periods.

1. <u>Pelvic Inflammatory Disease or P.I.D.</u>
The biggest risk with an IUD is the risk of getting P.I.D.. P.I.D. is an infection in your uterus and tubes. P.I.D. is very common. It is also very serious.

This is how an IUD can lead to an infection:

Normally, your uterus does not have germs in it. Any germs which are in your vagina cannot easily travel up into your uterus. However, when an IUD is in place, germs can get into your uterus. They can travel up the IUD string and into your uterus.

This is why the IUD is not a good choice for women who have many sexual partners. These partners may be carrying germs which can cause P.I.D.. An IUD is also not a good choice for women who have had P.I.D. before.

If P.I.D. is not treated, it can cause these serious problems:

- P.I.D. can cause scar tissue to build up in your tubes. This can make it impossible for you to ever get pregnant.

- P.I.D. can make you more likely to have tubal pregnancies. In a tubal pregnancy, the egg does not start to grow in your uterus (or womb). Instead, it starts to grow in one of your tubes. The egg cannot grow to full size in a tube. If you have a tubal pregnancy, then you will need to have an emergency operation to remove it. If you didn't have this operation, the tube would burst, and you could die.

- P.I.D. can cause severe long-term pain. (If you want to know more about P.I.D., please read p. 263, in Chapter 8, Sex.)

In the 1970's, many women were given an IUD called a Dalkon Shield. This kind of IUD caused many problems. Many women who had a Dalkon shield got Pelvic Inflammatory Disease, and many became sterile. If you have an IUD, ask your doctor to make sure that you don't have a Dalkon shield. If you do, have it removed right away.

You need to know the signs of P.I.D.. P.I.D. must be treated with antibiotics right away. Here are some signs of P.I.D. which you should look out for:

- pain in your lower abdomen (lower belly)
- unusual discharge from your vagina
- fever or chills drawing
- a feeling of being very sick, like the flu
- painful sex
- bleeding after sex
- pain in your back or legs
- pain when you pass urine (pee)
- bleeding from your vagina in between periods.

If you have any of these symptoms, go to your doctor at once.

2. Heavy Periods.

If you have an IUD, your periods may be heavier. If you lose a lot of blood every month, your blood may become low in iron. This is called being anemic. If you are anemic, you may feel run-down.

If you have very heavy periods, your doctor should test your blood to see if you are anemic. If you are anemic, then you need to eat more foods which contain iron. If you have lose a lot of blood every month, you may need to have your IUD removed.

These foods contain a lot of iron are:

- red meats
- leafy green vegetables
- peas and beans
- whole grain breads and cereals.

Because an IUD can cause health problems, you should have a medical check-up every year while you have one.

"How convenient is an IUD?"

An IUD is very convenient. Once it is in place, you only need to check for the string after every period. You should also check the string any time you have cramps.

A copper IUD must be replaced every two to three years. The kind which contain progesterone must be replaced every year.

"Where can I get an IUD?"

You can only get an IUD from a doctor.

Before you get an IUD, your doctor should ask you some questions about your medical history. If you have had any of the following problems, tell your doctor:

- P.I.D.
- bleeding between periods
- anemia
- miscarriages
- abnormal Pap tests
- heavy periods

If you have any of these problems, an IUD may not be the right birth control for you.

"How much does an IUD cost?"
An IUD costs from $35 to $83. Some birth control clinics put in IUDs for free

"Can I still get pregnant in the future if I use an IUD?"
An IUD <u>can</u> effect whether or not you can get pregnant in the future. An IUD can lead to P.I.D., and P.I.D. can make you unable to get pregnant again.

If you have only one sexual partner - and your partner has no other partners - you do not have a big risk of getting P.I.D.. However, if you have many partners, you have a much greater risk. If you want to have children in the future, and if you have many partners, an IUD is not the best method for you.

The Diaphragm

"What is a diaphragm?"
The diaphragm is a soft latex (rubber) cup. The diaphragm is placed at the back of your vagina. It covers your cervix which is the opening to your uterus (or womb). It must be used with a spermicidal jelly or cream. These jellies and creams kill sperm.

"How does a diaphragm work?"
The diaphragm is called a "barrier method" of birth control. The diaphragm is a barrier which blocks your cervix. This stops sperm from getting into your uterus.

The diaphragm also holds the spermicidal jelly in place over your cervix. The jelly kills any sperm which get around the edge of the diaphragm.

"How well does a diaphragm work?"
A diaphragm must fit you properly, and it must be used properly. It must be used every time you have intercourse.

Between 2 and 15 out of every 100 women who use a diaphragm get pregnant. Most of the women who get pregnant with this method have made a mistake in how they use their diaphragm.

"What is the right way to use the diaphragm?"

- Diaphragms come in several sizes. A trained doctor or a trained health worker needs to fit you for the right size.

- After you get fitted for a diaphragm, you must learn how to put it in. Before you leave the office, practise putting it in and taking it out. It should not be uncomfortable inside you. If it is uncomfortable, then it is the wrong size. If it causes cramps, or if it prevents you from peeing (passing urine), then it is the wrong size.

- After you put it in, check that it is in place. Insert two fingers inside your vagina, and feel your cervix. You should be able to feel that your cervix is covered by your diaphragm.

- You <u>must</u> use spermicidal jelly or cream with your diaphragm. Put one applicator-full of jelly inside the diaphragm before you insert it. The jelly is less active after about two hours. If you inserted jelly more than two hours before the man ejaculated, insert more jelly.

- If you have sex more than once, you need to insert more jelly. You need one applicator-full of jelly for each time the man ejaculates. However, you must not remove your diaphragm to do this. Instead, insert another full applicator of jelly into your vagina.

- You must leave your diaphragm in place for **eight hours** after your last intercourse. Don't take a bath or swim or douche during this time. Showers are OK.

- If you need a lubricant, use only the water-soluble kind. Never use Vaseline. Vaseline can make holes in your diaphragm.

- You need to take care of your diaphragm. After you remove it, wash it with warm water and then dry it very well. Check it for holes by holding it up to the light. If it is torn, you need a new one. Buy a new one at least every two years.

- You may need a new diaphragm if you gain or lose 10 pounds or more. You may need a new diaphragm if you have had an abortion, or a pregnancy, or surgery in your lower abdomen. If any of these has happened to you, ask your doctor to make sure your diaphragm still fits well.

"What are the risks to my health if I use a diaphragm?"
- Diaphragms are not harmful to your health.
- Some women are allergic to some spermicides. Some women are allergic to latex.
- Women who get a lot of bladder infections may get more infections if they use a diaphragm.
- If a pregnancy would be a serious risk to your health, then a diaphragm would not be the best birth control for you. This is because of the risk that you could get pregnant.

"How convenient is a diaphragm?"
Once you get used to a diaphragm, it's easy to use. Thousands of women use them. Some women put their diaphragm in every night. Then they don't have to worry about inserting it later if they need it.

"Where can I get a diaphragm?"
- You can get a diaphragm from your doctor or from a birth control clinic. Make sure your doctor, knows how to fit diaphragms.
- Make sure that the spermicidal jelly or cream you buy says "contraceptive" or "spermicidal" on the package. Make sure that you are not buying a "feminine hygiene" douche or perfume. These are useless for birth control. (They are just plain useless.) In some drug stores contraceptive jellies are kept near the feminine hygiene products. In others, they are near the condoms.

"How much does the diaphragm cost?"
Diaphragms cost about $28. You need a new one every one or two years.
Contraceptive jelly costs about $14 a tube. It contains enough jelly for about 12 applications.

"Can I still get pregnant in the future if I use a diaphragm?"
If you use a diaphragm, you will still be able to get pregnant in the future. If you do get pregnant, the jelly will not hurt the embryo.

Tubal Ligation.

"What is a tubal ligation?"
Tubal ligation is the operation which prevents you from getting pregnant ever again. It is often called "having your tubes tied". Tubal ligations are a permanent form of birth control.

"How does a tubal ligation work?"
During a tubal ligation, the tubes which carry the eggs are closed. This prevents the sperm from ever reaching an egg.

A tubal ligation is a simple operation. Nowadays, it is usually done as "day surgery". This means that you go in the morning, and you go home that evening. Most tubal ligations are done using an operation called a "laparoscopy".

In this operation, no large cuts are made. The doctor only makes two small cuts in your abdomen. One cut is near your navel (belly-button). The other cut is down near your hairline. Your tubes are closed off by burning them with an electrical current.

Your uterus will not be removed. You will still have periods. You may have menopause slightly earlier than other women do. Most women do not feel any different after they recover from the operation.

"How well does a tubal ligation work?"
Tubal ligations are nearly always successful. After a tubal ligation, only 2 women out of every <u>1000</u> will get pregnant. These women have the bad luck to have their tubes grow together again. This is very rare.

"What is the right way to use a tubal ligation?"
After the operation you can have intercourse without worrying about getting pregnant. You don't need to do anything else to prevent pregnancy.

"What are the risks to my health if I have a tubal ligation?"
The only risk is the risk of having an operation under a general anesthetic. Very few women have serious health problems after a tubal ligation.

However, a tubal ligation is slightly more dangerous than the sterilization operation for men. The operation for men is called a "vasectomy". It is done under a local anesthetic.

"How convenient is a tubal ligation?"
Tubal ligations are very convenient because you don't have to worry about ever getting pregnant again.

"Where can I get a tubal ligation?"
Ask your doctor to make an appointment for you with a gynecologist. A gynecologist is a doctor who specializes in health problems of women.

"How much does a tubal ligation cost?"
The cost of the operation is covered by the medical plan of your province.

"Can I still get pregnant in the future if I have a tubal ligation?"
Tubal ligation is a permanent method of birth control. After a tubal ligation you cannot get pregnant again.

Some women have tried to have their tubes connected again, but this is not easy. You need to have a long operation, and it is almost never a success. Have a tubal ligation only if you are sure that you don't want any more children.

Natural Family Planning.

"What is natural family planning?"
Natural family planning is not having intercourse when you can get pregnant. Natural family planning is also called "rhythm", "the calendar method", and "fertility awareness".

"How does natural family planning work?"
If you use this method, you must know when you are "fertile". You are "fertile" on the days when you can get pregnant. Once you know the days when you may be fertile, then you must not have intercourse on these days. Most women who use this method must avoid intercourse for about half of every month.

Natural family planning can be very difficult for women who do not have regular periods. This is because they don't know when they are going to be fertile. As a result, they must go without intercourse for long periods of time.

"How well does natural family planning work?"
Natural family planning is reliable only if you know how to use it very well. Between twenty and thirty of every 100 women who use this method get pregnant.

"What is the right way to use natural family planning?"

1. You have to learn to recognize "fertile" cervical mucus. This mucus is produced by your cervix when you are fertile.
2. You have to take your temperature every day. This will tell you when an egg is going to be released.
3. You have to keep a good record of your temperature, your cervical mucus, and of your periods.

It takes time and co-operation with your partner to learn how to use this method well.

If you want to use this method, you need to be taught how to use it. Ask your doctor or a birth control counsellor. It is a good idea to join a group or take a course to learn about it.

You need two things to make this method work well:
1. both you and your partner must be sure you want to use it,
2. both you and your partner must understand it very well.

"What are the risks to my health if I use natural family planning?"
The only risk is the risk of getting pregnant if you don't use the method correctly.

"How much does natural family planning cost?"
The thermometer costs about $10.

"Can I still get pregnant in the future if I natural family planning?"
This method will not affect whether or not you can get pregnant in the future.

(Some women have trouble getting pregnant. These women can get help from natural family planning. This method can teach them to notice when they are fertile. Then they can try to get pregnant at that time.)

Withdrawal.

"What is withdrawal?"
Withdrawal is a last resort method. It does **not** work very well. Many women who use it get pregnant. However, it is much better than nothing.

"How does withdrawal work?"
Withdrawal means that the man removes his penis from your vagina before he ejaculates. This is supposed to prevent sperm from getting into your vagina.

However, there are problems with this method:
- Some liquid comes out of the man's penis before he ejaculates, and this liquid also contains sperm.
- It is very hard for many men to know exactly when they are going to ejaculate. Sometimes they ejaculate before they want to.

"How well does withdrawal work?"
About 40 out of every 100 women who use it get pregnant. It is **not a good method** to depend on. However, it is better than nothing.

"What are the risks to my health if I use withdrawal?"
There are no health risks except the very big risk of getting pregnant.

Whichever method you choose, choose carefully. Find the safest and the most reliable birth control method for you.

Vaginal Infections

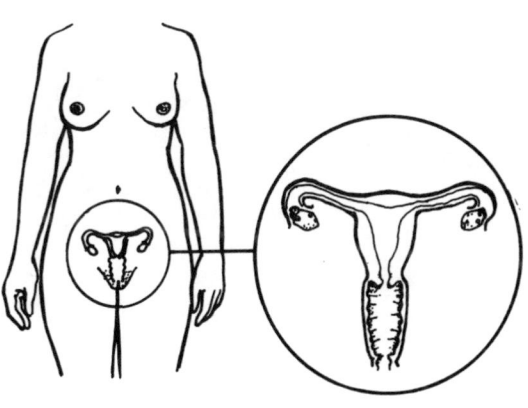

VAGINAL INFECTIONS

Most women get an infection in their vagina now and again. These infections are usually not serious, but they can be painful and annoying. Most infections can be prevented.

An infection in the vagina is also called a vaginal infection or vaginitis. One of the first signs of vaginitis is a change in the fluid which comes out of your vagina. This fluid is called vaginal discharge. It is important to know the difference between your normal vaginal discharge and an unusual discharge.

Here is a drawing which shows the parts of your body which I talk about in this chapter:

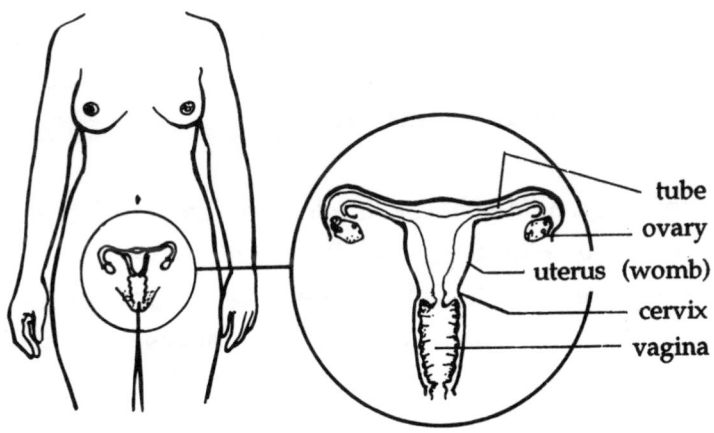

tube
ovary
uterus (womb)
cervix
vagina

Normal vaginal discharge.

There are two things to know about normal vaginal discharge:

(1) Every woman has some discharge from her vagina.

(2) Vaginal discharge always contains a balance of useful germs and harmful germs.

Vaginal discharge is normal and healthy. Some women have more than others. Pregnant women, women who have a new baby, and teenage girls often have much more discharge. This discharge can be inconvenient but it is normal. Notice how much you normally have.

Normal vaginal discharge comes from two places. The walls of your vagina produce part of it. The cervix, which is the opening of your uterus, produces the rest. Normal vaginal discharge is useful because it helps keep your vagina clean.

Normal vaginal discharge is clear or creamy white. It doesn't burn or itch, and it doesn't have an unpleasant smell. Check to see what yours normally looks and smells like. Then, if it changes, you will know that you might have an infection.

You may notice a few days of heavier discharge. This happens about two weeks before your period. This special discharge is clear and slippery, and it looks like raw egg white. It is produced during the time when you can get pregnant, that is, when you are "fertile". It is called "fertile mucus".

This mucus is produced by your cervix. It can be very useful. At the time of the month when you can get pregnant, it helps the sperm travel up into your uterus. At other times it helps keep germs out of the uterus. It also contains a mild acid which stops harmful germs from growing well.

Your discharge always contains bacteria and other germs. Some of them are useful, and others can be harmful. Normally there is a balance between all of these germs. When they are in balance, the harmful germs are not able to grow in large amounts. When this balance is changed, the harmful ones can start to grow in large amounts. This can cause a vaginal infection.

Unusual vaginal discharge.

There are several different kinds of unusual discharges.

- Some unusual discharges look different. Some are thick and white, and look a bit like cottage cheese. Others are yellowish, greenish or grey.
- Some unusual discharges smell different.
- Some unusual discharges cause burning or itching. They cause sores or bumps on the outer lips of your vagina, or on the inside of your vagina. Your outer lips may become redder than usual and sore to touch.
- Some unusual discharges are hard to see. However, you know they are there because sex is painful.

"What does an unusual discharge mean?"
An unusual discharge will mean one of three things:
(1) Most often it means you have a simple vaginal infection.
(2) Sometimes it means that your cervix or your vagina is irritated but you do not have an infection.
(3) Sometimes an unusual discharge means that you have a Sexually Transmitted Disease (STD). Sexually Transmitted Diseases used to be called VD.

Gonorrhea and chlamydia are common STDs. (If you want more information on STDs, please read p. 246, in Chapter 8, Sex.)

STDs can be very serious. These diseases are caught from a sexual partner. The infection starts in your vagina or your cervix. Then it can travel up into your uterus (or womb) and into your tubes. When the infection is in your uterus or tubes, it is called Pelvic Inflammatory Disease, or P.I.D.. If you have P.I.D., you can end up unable to get pregnant. You might also have many tubal pregnancies, or be in severe pain for months or even years.

If you have a new discharge, and a new sexual partner, **go to your doctor.**
If you have burning when you pee (when you pass urine), and a new sexual partner, **go to your doctor.**

Only a pelvic examination and a lab test will show for sure what kind of infection you have.
If you want more information about P.I.D., please read p. 263, in Chapter 8, Sex.

Check with your doctor

Common Vaginal Infections.

An unusual discharge usually means that you have a vaginal infection. A vaginal infection is not something to be ashamed of. It does not mean that you are not clean. Vaginal infections are very common. Most women get them now and again.

Most vaginal infections are not serious, but they can be very annoying. The common vaginal infections are caused by yeast, trichomonas or gardnerella.

Yeast Infections.

(Yeast infections are also called thrush, candidiasis and monilia.)

"What is it?"
- Yeast is found in small amounts in a healthy vagina.
- It only causes an infection when it grows in large amounts.
- Yeast infections are very common.

"How will I know if I have it?"

- The discharge from a yeast infection is white or cream-coloured. It often looks like cottage cheese. It may smell like the yeast used in bread.
- If you have a yeast infection, you will likely feel burning or itching. The itching may be very strong.
- Your outer vaginal lips may be swollen and red and sore to touch.
- Sex may be painful.

"What causes it?"

- Yeast is present in your vagina all the time. You will get a yeast infection when the normal balance in your vagina is changed. This change allows the yeast to grow.
- This yeast is like bread-yeast. It can grow well whenever it is warm, moist, and well-fed with sugar.
- There are three common ways to allow the yeast to grow:
  - Yeast will grow if you make the area warm and moist. This can happen if you wear clothes that don't allow the area around the opening of your vagina to breathe.
  - Yeast will grow if you remove the yeast's natural "enemies". This can happen if you take antibiotics, or if you douche often.

- Yeast will grow if the cells in your vagina contain too much sugar. This can happen if you eat a lot of sugar. It can also happen if you are pregnant, or if you are on the Pill, or if you are diabetic.

"How can I get rid of it?"
- Sometimes you can get rid of a minor yeast infection by wearing looser clothes.
- However, if you have a serious infection, you will likely need medicine to get rid of it.
- Your doctor will likely give you a prescription for some medicine containing nystatin. It is available in creams, suppositories, and also in special tampons. It is important that you use these medicines correctly. Check with your doctor or druggist if you are not sure how to use yours. If the medicine does not get rid of your infection, you may have two kinds of infection at the same time.
- You can do some things yourself to relieve the pain and itching. You can add some vinegar to your bath water. You can also apply watered-down vinegar to your outer vaginal lips, by using a wash cloth or cotton ball. Use about one teaspoon of vinegar in one cup of water. This is very soothing **unless** you have a serious infection with open sores.

- After you have got rid of your infection, read the list of ways to prevent infections on p. 330. Then you may never have to worry about getting a yeast infection again.
- Some women use herbs to get rid of vaginal infections. If you are interested, you will have to track down someone who knows about herbal remedies. You could ask a women's health centre, an acupuncturist, or a holistic health centre. Even though herbal remedies can be useful, your doctor may not support this kind of treatment.

Trichomonas Infections.

(Trichomonas is pronounced trick-a-MO-nas. It is sometimes called "trick".)

"What is it?"

- Trichomonas is a common vaginal infection caused by a germ which is passed from one person to another. It is annoying, but it is usually not dangerous.

"How will I know if I have it?"

- Trichomonas can produce a lot of yellowish green or grey discharge which has a foul odour.
- The outer lips of your vagina may be red and tender. Inside your vagina you may feel itchy and sore. You may feel like you have to pass urine (pee) more often. It may be painful when you do.
- You may have trichomonas without knowing it. A male partner may have some signs of it, such as discharge or burning when he passes urine.

"What causes it?"

- Usually trichomonas is passed from one person to another during sex.
- Sometimes it is passed on by sharing wet bathing suits, wet towels or face cloths, or from toilet seats.

"How do I get rid of it?"

- A trichomonas infection usually won't go away on its own. You need to get a prescription for it.
- First, your doctor will examine you. Usually the doctor will take a sample of your discharge. This sample, which is called a "smear", is then sent to a lab. The workers in the lab will report to your doctor if there is trichomonas in the smear.
- If you do have trichomonas, you will get a drug called metronidazole. It is commonly called Flagyl, and it is given as suppositories or pills. Doctors usually give people a prescription for 3 to 7 days. Some doctors have found that a 1-day dose works just about as well. Ask your doctor about this.

- Flagyl is a strong drug which has several side effects when it is taken as pills. It can cause nausea, headaches, cramps, and diarrhea. So, only take Flagyl after the smear proves you have trichomonas.
- Take Flagyl pills with food so it won't upset your stomach. Don't drink any alcohol while you are taking Flagyl. Don't drink any alcohol until two days after your prescription is finished. Alcohol plus Flagyl can make you sick.
- Your sexual partner must take the drug too. Then you won't pass the infection back and forth. If you are not too sore to have intercourse, use condoms until you are both cured.
- If you are taking medicine for trichomonas, you may end up with a yeast infection in your vagina. This is because the drug kills off the yeast's natural "enemies". Be sure to read the section above on Yeast Infections, and do what you can to prevent another infection.

Gardnerella Infections.

(Gardnerella is pronounced gard-ner-EL-la.)

"What is it?"
- Gardnerella used to be called Hemophilus. Sometimes it is hard to diagnose. It is often the cause of an infection which doctors call "non-specific vaginitis".

"How will I know if I have it?"
- You may have it without knowing it, and it may be giving you no trouble.
- If you do have a discharge, it will be white, grey, or yellow. Often it has an unpleasant, fishy smell.
- Your vagina and vaginal lips may be sore.
- Intercourse may be painful.

"What causes it?"
- You may have caught it by having sex with a person who has it.
- It can happen if the balance in your vagina changes. This change can allow the gardnerella germ to grow in larger numbers.

"How do I get rid of it?"
- Usually doctors will give you and your partner either a drug called Flagyl, or an antibiotic, or a sulfa drug. Flagyl is given as suppositories or pills. Flagyl is a strong drug which can cause side effects when it is taken as pills. It can cause nausea, headaches, cramps, and diarrhea.
- Take Flagyl pills with food so it won't upset your stomach. Don't drink any alcohol while you are taking Flagyl. Don't drink any alcohol until two days after your prescription is finished. Alcohol plus Flagyl can make you sick.
- If you are not too sore to have sex, use condoms until you are both cured.

Less Common Vaginal Infections.

Some vaginal infections have other causes:
- **Allergies.**
  Sometimes vaginitis is caused by an allergy to a soap or vaginal spray. It can also be caused by perfumed menstrual pads and by coloured or perfumed toilet paper. This kind of vaginitis will go away when you stop using whatever is irritating you.
- **A forgotten tampon.**
  Sometimes a discharge is caused by a forgotten tampon, which needs to be removed.

- **Menopause.**
  Some vaginitis is caused by the hormone changes of menopause. Women who are going through menopause have less of the hormone called estrogen. Less estrogen can make your vagina drier and less stretchable. Your vagina may also be slower to become lubricated (or wet) during sex. Intercourse may become painful. Your vagina and outer lips may be itchy and sore. If your vagina is irritated, it can become infected more easily. Many women get more yeast infections during menopause.

  These infections can be prevented. Please read
  p. 330 in this chapter.

- **Toxic Shock Syndrome.**
  Toxic Shock Syndrome (TSS) is another kind of infection which can begin in your vagina. TSS is very serious, however it is also very rare. Very few women get TSS.

  TSS is caused by bacteria. The bacteria start to grow in your vagina. Then they can travel into your blood. After the bacteria gets into your blood, they can make you extremely sick. They can even kill you.

Most women who get TSS are using a tampon at the time. If you have TSS, you will get a sudden high fever, and vomiting or diarrhea. You may also get a rash.

If you are using a tampon, and you begin to feel like you have a very bad flu, you may have TSS. Remove your tampon and use a pad instead. Then call your doctor or go to a hospital right away. TSS must be treated very quickly.

If you want to avoid getting TSS:
- Wash your hands before using a tampon.
- Change your tampon every 4 to 6 hours.
- Use a pad at night instead of a tampon.

How to Prevent Vaginal Infections.

Vaginal infections are caused three different ways:
(1) Some vaginal infections are caused by changes in the normal balance in your vagina.
(2) Some vaginal infections are caused by germs.
(3) Some vaginal infections are caused by hormone changes.
There are different ways to prevent each kind of vaginitis.

(1) **How to prevent vaginal infections caused by changes in the normal conditions in your vagina.**

When the normal balance in your vagina is changed, harmful germs can begin to grow. These germs are already living in your vagina. If too many of them have a chance to grow, they cause an infection.

Here are some ways to prevent infections which are caused by changing the balance in your vagina. If you do these things, you will keep a normal balance in your vagina:

- Avoid clothes which keep the area around the opening of your vagina warm and moist. When it is warm and moist, it is a perfect place for yeast to grow. Avoid pantyhose and nylon or synthetic underpants. Avoid very tight jeans, and don't wear nylons under jeans.
- Wear cotton underpants. Don't wear a mini pad every day. Wear panty-hose with a ventilated crotch or a cotton crotch. Cotton absorbs moisture and lets the vaginal area stay dry. If you still get a lot of yeast infections, try wearing a garter belt and stockings instead of panty-hose.
- Wear shirts or night gowns to bed. Don't wear pajamas.

- Don't use strong, perfumed soaps, or bath oils, or bubble baths. They change the natural acids in your vagina. This allows harmful bacteria and yeast to grow more easily. Little girls can also get vaginal infections from using bubble baths.

- Don't use vaginal deodorant sprays. They are often very strong. They can burn and cause itching and discharge. We all have a natural odour. If you have an unpleasant odour, then you may have an infection. It needs to be treated, not covered up.

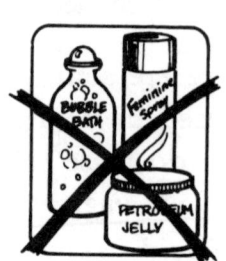

- Don't use coloured or perfumed toilet paper. Don't use deodorant tampons or menstrual pads. Both the perfume and the dyes can burn your skin. Many women are allergic to coloured toilet paper.

- Don't douche. Douching is a way of spraying water into your vagina to clean it. Douching is an old-fashioned idea. You do not need to douche. Your vagina does not need to be "cleaned out", because it cleans itself.

Besides being unnecessary, douching can also cause problems:

1. Douching upsets the natural balance of your vagina. This can cause vaginal infections.

2. Douching is useless for birth control. In fact, it can even help to make you pregnant! This is because douching can force some of the sperm up into your uterus.

3. Douching can be dangerous if it forces liquid up into your uterus. This can cause an infection in your uterus.

- Don't have sex if your vagina is dry. Don't have sex if you have an infection and you are sore. If you want a lubricating jelly, use one that dissolves in water such as KY jelly. You can buy it in a drug store.
Don't use petroleum jelly such as Vaseline. It does not dissolve in water, so it can trap harmful germs in your vagina. It can also weaken condoms and diaphragms.

- Cut down on the amount of sugar you eat. The sugar in sweet foods and in alcohol builds up in the cells in your body. The yeast lives off this sugar.

- Don't take antibiotics unless you are sure you need them. If you have to take an antibiotic, you may end up with a vaginal infection. This is because antibiotics upset the normal balance in your vagina. They kill off both harmful bacteria and useful bacteria, everywhere in your body. The useful bacteria prevent yeast from growing very well. When these useful bacteria are killed off, the yeast can grow in large numbers, causing an infection.

If you need to take an antibiotic, remember the ways to help prevent infections which are listed on these pages. Also, try eating plain yogurt while they are taking the antibiotic. Yogurt contains some of the useful bacteria. Yogurt can help to prevent both yeast infections and diarrhea.

(2) How to prevent vaginal infections caused by germs which are not usually found in your vagina.

Here are some ways to prevent infections caused by new germs:

- Wash or have a bath every day. Wear clean underwear.
- Don't share towels, washcloths, or bathing suits with others.

- After you've gone to the toilet, always wipe from the front to the back. You don't want any germs from your anus to get into your vagina.
- If you have anal sex, be sure your partner's penis is clean before it goes into your vagina. To be safe, your partner should wear a condom. Then remove it before you have vaginal intercourse.

(3) How to prevent vaginal infections caused by hormone changes.

Hormones are chemicals which are produced by your body. The amount of hormone in your body is called the hormone level.

Pregnancy, breast-feeding, birth control pills, menopause, hysterectomy and diabetes all cause changes in hormone levels. A change in a hormone level can affect your body in many ways. One result can be a vaginal infection.

Here are some ways to prevent vaginal infections which are caused by changes in hormone levels:

- **Birth Control Pills and Pregnancy.**
Both birth control pills and pregnancy raise the hormone level in your body. This causes the cells in your vagina to hold more sugar. This sugar is food for the yeast.

To prevent yeast infections, keep the area around your vagina dry, and eat less sugar. If you get a lot of infections while you are on the Pill, you may need a different Pill, or a different kind of birth control.

• Menopause.

During menopause, your hormone levels drop. As a result, your vagina may become drier on the inside. When it is dry, it can get irritated and infected. Here are three ways to prevent infections during menopause:

- Use a lubricating jelly, such as K-Y jelly. You can buy lubricating jellies in a drug store. Choose one which can dissolve in water. Do not use petroleum jelly, such as Vaseline.

- Making love can also help this problem, as long as it doesn't hurt. Making love or masturbating can help to make your vagina more able to lubricate itself.

- If a lubricant doesn't work, estrogen creams can help. Estrogen cream is not used as a lubricant before sex. You need to put some in your vagina every day. After a couple of weeks, your vagina will likely be more comfortable.
Then you only need to use the cream a few times a week. You need a prescription for estrogen cream.

Extra estrogen is not safe for all woman. [If you are interested, you can read more about estrogen in the section called Taking Hormones on p. 392, in Chapter 13, <u>Menopause</u>.]

• **Diabetes.**
People with diabetes are more likely to get infections. This is because diabetes causes the cells to hold more sugar. If you often get vaginal infections, make sure that you follow your special diet. Also, keep the outer vaginal area dry and follow the other rules for preventing infections on p. 330.

What to do if you get an infection.

If you remember these rules, you will be able to prevent most vaginal infections. However, you may get one now and again, no matter how careful you are.

If you know an infection is starting, you may be able to stop it before it is serious. You may be able to remove the cause if it is something like a new soap or nylon panties.

However, if you can't get rid of it, don't put up with it. See your doctor. While you are treating your infection, learn how to prevent it from happening again.

Getting help from your doctor.

The better your doctor can see your discharge, the easier it is to know what is causing it. You can do some things to make it easier for your doctor to clearly see your discharge.

- Before you go to your doctor:
  - Do not douche. You can have a shower or a bath.
  - Do not use a vaginal deodorant spray.
  - Do not use old medicine left over from another infection.
  - Do not use contraceptive foam. Use another kind of birth control instead.
- Don't make an appointment during your period. The blood makes it very hard for the doctor to clearly see your discharge.
- Be ready to describe the infection to your doctor. If you have had a new sexual partner, tell her or him. You could have caught something from your partner.
- The doctor may have to do some laboratory tests to find out what is causing your infection.
  To do the test, the doctor will take a sample of your vaginal discharge. This sample is sent to a laboratory. There they figure out which germ is causing the problem.

- If your doctor gives you medicine for your infection, be sure to take the full prescription. You may feel much better after the second day, but keep taking it. If you take it all, you can be almost sure that the drug has killed all the germs.

Ask your doctor if you need to have another test after you've finished taking the medicine. Ask your doctor if your partner should get some medicine too. If she or he is not treated, then you can pass the infection back and forth. If you have a male partner, be sure he uses condoms until you are cured.

Before you leave your doctor, be sure you find out:
1. what kind of infection you have.
2. what caused the infection.
3. how to get rid of it.
4. how to prevent it from happening again.

You should be able to avoid most vaginal infections. If you do get an infection, try to figure out what kind you have. If you know the kind, you might be able to get rid of it on your own. You might be able to remove what is causing it.

It you can't get rid of it, see your doctor. Learn what caused it, and learn how to prevent it from happening again.

Pap Tests

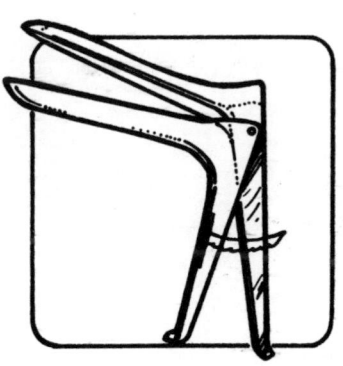

PAP TESTS

What Pap tests are for.

Pap tests are an easy way to find out if you have cancer in your cervix. The cervix is the opening to your uterus (or womb).

Why Pap tests are important.

Cancer of the cervix, or "cervical cancer", is fairly common. It usually grows very slowly. If it is found early and removed, cervical cancer can nearly always be cured.

When cervical cancer is just starting to grow, you will not know it is there. Cervical cancer doesn't cause any pain or discharge for many years. This is why some women don't know they have it until it is too late. This is why some women die of it every year. Pap tests could have prevented most of these deaths. Pap tests would have found the cancer before it had time to spread.

A Pap test is usually done during an internal (or vaginal) examination. Many women feel embarrassed having an internal examination so they avoid them. If you feel embarrassed, remind yourself that Pap tests are a necessary part of keeping healthy. You owe it to yourself to have a regular Pap test.

How often you should have a Pap test.

Pap tests once a year.
Many doctors do a Pap test as part of your yearly check-up. Since the test is so easy and safe, this seems like a very good idea.

- You should start having a yearly Pap test when you become 18, or when you start having sex, whichever comes first.

- You should continue having a Pap test every year for the next five years.

- If you have had many years of normal Pap tests, you are likely in less danger of getting cervical cancer. After five years of normal Pap tests, some doctors suggest a Pap test only every two or three years. Other doctors suggest a Pap test every year, just to be safe.

- Doctors do not agree on how often you should have a Pap test after your menopause. Some doctors suggest a Pap test every year. Some say every three years. Some say every five years.

- If you have had a hysterectomy because of cancer, then you should have a Pap test every year for the rest of your life. (After a hysterectomy, a Pap test is done by testing some cells from your vagina. If your cervix was not removed in the operation, then some cells are also taken from it.)

Pap tests every six months.

Some women need a Pap test every six months because they have more risk of getting cervical cancer.

- Women with venereal warts, and women with herpes may be more likely to get cervical cancer. Venereal warts and herpes are sexually transmitted diseases.

- Women whose mothers took D.E.S. may be more likely to get cervical cancer.

  D.E.S. stands for Di-ethyl-stilbestrol. D.E.S. is a drug which contains estrogen. It was used between 1941 and 1971. Doctors gave it to pregnant women because it was supposed to prevent miscarriages.

  Now we know that D.E.S. caused health problems for some of the babies of these women. These problems don't show up until the people are teenagers or adults.

Women whose mothers took D.E.S. are called "D.E.S. daughters". D.E.S. daughters may have trouble getting pregnant. They may have more miscarriages, and more problems with their menstrual periods. A small number of D.E.S. daughters get cancer of the vagina and the cervix.

If you were born between 1941 and 1971, try to find out if your mother took D.E.S.. Ask her if she took any pills, or had any shots, to prevent a miscarriage. It may be hard to find out what drugs she took. She may not remember, and her medical records may have been destroyed.

If you think you are a D.E.S. daughter, you need to be examined by a doctor who has experience with D.E.S.. The doctor will look for any problems which may have been caused by the D.E.S..

- Women who have had cervical cancer once are more likely to get it again.

- Women who have many male sexual partners are more likely to get cervical cancer.

- Women who are heavy smokers are more likely to get cervical cancer.

- Women who work with cancer-causing chemicals are more likely to get cervical cancer. Women whose husbands work with cancer-causing chemicals are also more likely to get cervical cancer.

How a Pap test is done.

In a Pap test, your doctor takes a sample of cells from your cervix. Then the cells are sent to a laboratory to be examined for cancer.

First the doctor puts a speculum into your vagina. The speculum holds the walls of your vagina open. Here is a drawing of a speculum:

Using the speculum, the doctor will find your cervix.

In the drawing on the next page you can see that your cervix is at the inner end of your vagina. The cervix is the neck of your uterus (or womb). It is the opening to your uterus. Menstrual blood flows out through your cervix. Sperm can travel up through the cervix into your uterus. Your cervix can also open (or dilate) to allow a baby to pass through.

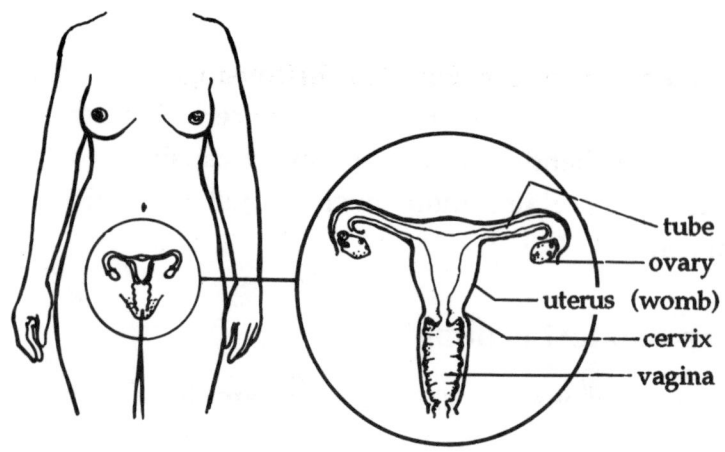

The doctor will examine your cervix to look for anything unusual such as an infection or warts.

Then the doctor will take a scraping of cells from the centre of your cervix. To do this, the doctor will use a small stick shaped like this:

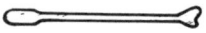

The stick is placed in the centre of your cervix. Then it is twirled around to get a good sample of cells. These cells are smeared onto a slide. (This is why Pap tests are sometimes called Pap "smears"). Then the slide is sent to a medical laboratory to be tested.

This drawing shows a Pap test being done:

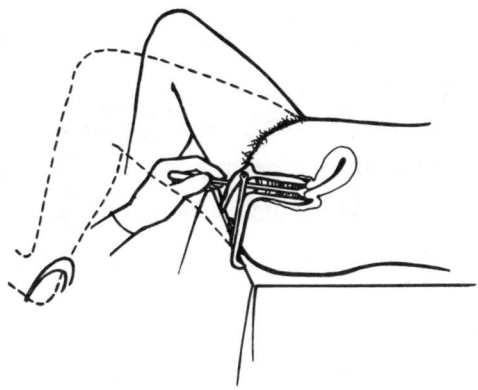

Pap tests are painless for most women. They only take a few minutes to do.

It is important for the doctor to get a good clean sample of cells.

- Don't use contraceptive foam either the night or morning before your Pap test. The foam may cover your cervix. This makes it harder to get a good sample of cells.
- Don't douche beforehand. Douching can remove some of the cells. Baths and swimming are OK.
- Don't have a Pap test while you have your period. The blood makes it hard for the doctor to get a good sample of cells.

What the test results mean.

After a few days, the laboratory will send the test results to your doctor.

- If your cells are normal, you likely won't hear anything from your doctor. So, with a Pap test, "No news is good news". If you want to be sure, call your doctor after a week, and ask for your Pap test results.
- If there are some **abnormal** (not normal) cells, your doctor will let you know. If you have abnormal cells, your doctor will likely want to repeat the test. Then they can see if the results are the same both times. (An abnormal Pap test result is sometimes called a "positive" test.)

Try not to worry if you hear that you have abnormal cells. **Abnormal cells do not always mean cancer.** Abnormal cells mean many different things:

1. Abnormal cells could mean that you have an infection. If you do, you need to have it treated. Then you need to have another Pap test after the infection is gone.

2. Abnormal cells could mean that your cervix has some unusual - but not dangerous - cells. Often these abnormal cells will become normal after a few months.

3. Abnormal cells could mean that your cervix has some precancerous cells. Precancerous means that they may become cancer at a later time. Usually they are slow to become cancerous.

4. Abnormal cells could mean that there are cancer cells in your cervix. Remember: most cervical cancer can be cured.

What happens if you have abnormal cells in your cervix.

The kind of treatment you need depends on the kind of abnormal cells you have.

1. Infected Cells.

If you have abnormal cells because of an infection, you will need to have it treated. Your sexual partners may need to be treated also.

2. Unusual Cells Which Are Not Precancerous.

If you have abnormal cells which are unusual, your doctor will likely want to wait for a few months. Then you will need another Pap test to see if anything has changed.

If the second Pap test shows that the abnormal cells have gone, then there is no problem. Your doctor may tell you to have another Pap test in 6 months. If the abnormal cells are still there, your doctor will likely want to know more about the cells. The doctor will likely treat them as if they were precancerous cells.

3. Precancerous Cells.

If you have precancerous cells, it can be hard to know what is the best thing to do. This is because often abnormal cells become normal again, without any treatment. Also, cancer of the cervix is usually slow-growing. You usually have time to think, and to make your decision carefully. In the meantime, you should have regular Pap tests to know if the cells are changing.

Some doctors are doing research to figure out how abnormal cells can become normal again. Sometimes this happens because the woman had an infection when she had the Pap test done. When the infection was cured, the cells became normal again.

Some research is trying to find out if condoms can protect the cervix. In one test, nearly all the women who used condoms during sex found that their abnormal cells become normal again. This happened after five or six months of using condoms. Other research is looking at the effects of eating well and getting rid of stress.

So, you can usually go slowly. You may be able to get rid of your abnormal cells without having any surgery. Find out as much as you can about your problem. Then you and your doctor can decide together what to do.

To help you and your doctor decide, you both will likely want to know more about your abnormal cells. To find out more, you will likely be asked to go for "colposcopy" and a "punch biopsy".

Colposcopy and Punch Biopsy.
Colposcopy is a way for doctors to get an enlarged view of the abnormal cells in your cervix. To do this, they use a colposcope — an instrument with a magnifying lens and a powerful light.

After looking at your abnormal cells with the colposcope, the doctor will take a sample of the cells. This sample of cells is called a "biopsy". The doctor uses an instrument like a paper punch, so this biopsy is called a "punch biopsy". Then the cells are sent to a laboratory where they are examined.

The results of the colposcopy and the punch biopsy will help you and your doctor decide what to do next.

(a) If you had a very small area of precancerous cells, you may not need any more treatment. You will need to have another Pap test after 6 months.

(b) If you have a slightly larger area of precancerous cells, then you likely should have them removed. This is usually easy to do. The cells can usually be removed in a doctor's office, or in an out-patient clinic.

There are two methods for removing small areas of cells:
- The cells may be destroyed by freezing them.
- The cells may be destroyed by using a laser on them.

These methods can be painful and unpleasant. Ask your doctor what treatment you are going to have. Also find out what to expect afterwards.

(c) If you have an even larger area of precancerous cells, then you will have to have surgery in a hospital. This operation is called a "cone biopsy". A cone-shaped section of your cervix is removed. Your cervix and uterus do not have to be removed to remove the cells. After you recover, you should still be able to get pregnant, and have a normal pregnancy.

4. Cancer Cells.
If you have abnormal cells which are cancer cells, it may be easy to remove them. It depends on whether or not the cancer has spread.

(a) Cancer in situ.
If the cancer cells are only in the outer layers of your cervix, then this cancer is completely curable. This cancer is called "cancer in situ", or cancer which has not spread.

If the cancer has not spread, only the area of cancer cells needs to be removed. This is done either by the freezing treatment or the laser treatment. Sometimes a cone biopsy is necessary.

Some doctors also suggest a hysterectomy, unless you want more children. (A hysterectomy is an operation which removes your uterus, including your cervix. You should not need to have your ovaries removed.)

This operation definitely prevents cervical cancer from starting again. However, a hysterectomy is a major operation. It shouldn't be done without a very good reason. If you want more information about hysterectomy, please read p. 399 in Chapter 13, <u>Menopause</u>.

(b) Invasive Cancer.

The cancer may have started to spread. This cancer is called "invasive", because it "invades" or spreads. The cancer may have spread deeper into your cervix or up into your uterus.

If the cancer has spread, a hysterectomy is usually done. Radiation and drug treatment may also be necessary, depending on how far the cancer has spread.

If you have abnormal cells on your cervix, remember this:

1) Try to get as much information as possible. This way you and your doctor can make the best decision together.

2) Remember that you have the right to a second opinion. If you are confused or unhappy about the treatment which your doctor has suggested, you can talk with another doctor. Try to find one who has experience in treating cervical cancer. Together, you and your doctor can find the best treatment for you.

Cancer of the cervix can almost always be cured if it is found early.

Do yourself a favour: have a regular Pap test and be safe.

Examining
Your Breasts

12

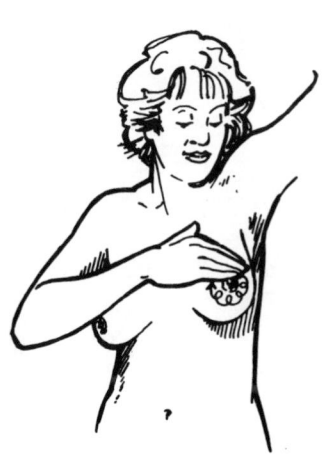

EXAMINING YOUR BREASTS

Checking your breasts every month is a good way to take care of yourself.

Most of us know that we should examine our breasts every month - but many of us don't do it. Some of us are afraid that we might find a lump, and that the lump might be cancer. Some of us are afraid that a lump means that we will lose a breast. Some of us are shy about touching our breasts. Some of us just never get around to doing it. Some of us think our breasts belong to our babies, or to our husbands, instead of to ourselves.

Why you should examine your breasts.

Breast cancer is the largest cause of death in women who are between ages 37 and 55. One out of every ten woman in Canada will get breast cancer. However, many will not die from it. One way to protect yourself is to find the cancer before it has spread. If it is found early, breast cancer is much easier to cure.

Some cancer can be cured and some cannot. For the cancer which can be cured, the earlier you find it the better.

Breast self-examination is easy to do well. You are the best person to do it because:

- You know your own breasts best.
- You can know what is normal for them and what isn't.
- You can know your own breasts better than your doctor who only examines them once a year.

Every woman should make a habit of checking her breasts once each month. Every woman means teenagers, pregnant women, breast-feeding mothers, middle-aged women, older women, and you.

When to examine your breasts.

You need to examine your breasts once a month. It's easy to remember if you do it at the same time each month. Many women check their breasts every month when their period ends. This is a good time because at the end of your period your breasts aren't tender to touch.

Some women don't have periods because of menopause, a hysterectomy, pregnancy or certain drugs. If you don't have periods, then pick the same day to check your breasts every month. Choose a day that will be easy to remember such as the first day of every month. Check your breasts on the same day each month so you won't forget.

How to examine your breasts.

Examining your breasts is easy. You need to examine them in two ways: by looking at them and by feeling them.

The Looking Part.

1. Sit or stand in front of a mirror with your arms relaxed at your sides.
Look for any changes in the size or shape of your breasts. Look for any rash, or puckering, or dimpling of your skin. Look for any change in your nipples.
Look for any discharge or fluid leaking from your nipples.

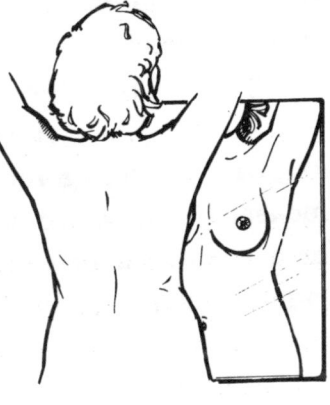

2. Move your arms up and down. Lift both of your arms over your head. See if any part of either breast doesn't move as easily as it used to. See if any part of one breast doesn't move as easily as that part of the other breast.

Remember that both breasts never look exactly the same. However, if you notice that one looks very different from the other, have this checked by a doctor. If you notice that one breast looks more different than usual, have this checked by a doctor.

The Feeling Part.

When you are feeling your breasts, do not use your fingertips. Your finger tips are too sensitive. If you use them, you will feel lots of normal lumps and bumps. These lumps and bumps are not cancer. They are milk glands and fat. If you use your finger tips, you may get worried for nothing.

Instead of your finger tips, you need to hold your fingers together. Keep your fingers together and use the flat part about an inch and a half from your finger tips.

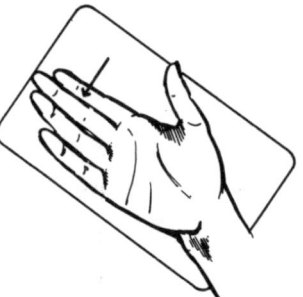

You will be feeling for a single, hard lump or thickening. Some women say that it is like looking for a bean in a bag of rice. You will be pressing your breast gently but firmly against your chest.

The steps to follow when you feel your breasts.
The best way to examine your breasts is lying down.
This is very important if you have large breasts.
When you are lying down, it is easier to reach the
under parts of your breast. Some women with
smaller breasts examine them in the bath or shower.
The soap and water make it easy to do. Choose the
way that works for you. Whichever way you choose,
be sure that you do each of these steps.

Step 1. Start with your left breast. Lie on your bed
with a pillow under your left shoulder. Put your
left hand under your head.

Keeping the fingers of
your right hand together,
press your breast against
your chest. Move your
fingers in little circles.
Start at the outside of
your breast, near your
armpit. Feel slowly and
carefully all the way
around the outside rim of
your breast.

Step 2. Now, move your fingers closer to your nipple. Feel all the way around again. Repeat this until you are sure you have covered your whole breast and nipple.

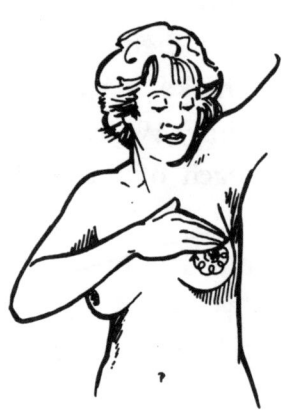

Step 3. Squeeze your nipple. If you are not pregnant or breast-feeding, you should not have any discharge. If you have a discharge, tell your doctor. A discharge is usually harmless but it should be checked.

(If you are pregnant, the only discharge from your breasts should be colostrum. Colostrum is the creamy liquid which comes before breast milk. If you are breast-feeding, the only discharge from your breasts should be breast milk.)

Step 4. Then lower your arm to your side. Carefully feel your armpit. This step is very important. Breast tissue is also found under your arm, and some breast cancers start there.

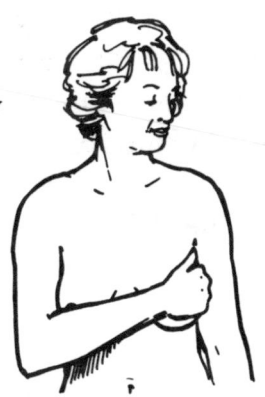

Step 5. Do the same examination on your other breast and armpit. Both your breasts should feel about the same. If they don't, ask your doctor to check them.

These five steps should take you about 10 minutes, once a month. Remember, you're worth it!!

Breast Lumps.

If you find a lump or a change in your breast, ask your doctor to check it right away. Most lumps are not cancer. Only one out of every nine or ten lumps is cancer.

Your doctor may tell you that your breast lump is called a "cyst". Cysts are not cancer, and they are usually harmless. They may swell up a bit every month before your period, and go down after. Remember where yours normally are. Then you will know the difference between a cyst and a new lump. If you are not sure, ask your doctor to check it for you.

Some lumps are caused by cancer. Nowadays there are several different ways to treat breast cancer. In the past, many women had their whole breast removed. This operation is called a Mastectomy. Nowadays, it is much more common to have only the lump removed. This operation is called a Lumpectomy. Most women also have radiation treatment.

If your doctor suggests an operation, get a second opinion from a cancer specialist, or a breast specialist. Find out all you can before you make up your mind.

"Who will get breast cancer?"

Doctors cannot say exactly who will or who won't get cancer. However, they know that some women are more likely to get it than others.

If you are more likely to get breast cancer, doctors say that you are in a **high-risk group** for breast cancer. The women in this list are in a **high-risk group** for breast cancer:

- Women who have had breast cancer before.
- Women who eat a lot of fatty food.
- Women who have a mother or a sister who had breast cancer before they were 40 years old.
- Women who have had a lot of X-rays.
- Women who took D.E.S.. D.E.S. stands for Di-ethyl-stilbestrol. D.E.S. is a harmful drug which was given to some pregnant women between 1941 and 1971. (If you want to know more about D.E.S., please read p. 343 in Chapter 11, Pap Tests.)

If your mother took D.E.S., or if you have taken estrogen during menopause, you may also have a higher risk of getting breast cancer.

Your doctor may ask you questions to find out if you are in a high-risk group. If you are, it does not mean that you will get breast cancer for sure. It does mean that you should be very careful to examine your breasts every month. You should also eat less foods which contain fat, and you should not take estrogen.

If you are in a high-risk group, your doctor might send you for a mammogram.

Mammograms.

A mammogram is a painless way of getting a picture of the inside of your breast, using a low dose of X-rays. There are two reasons for using mammograms:

(1) Mammograms are used if a woman has a lump which can be felt. These mammograms give the doctor more information about the lump.

If you have a lump, your doctor will likely want to do a biopsy. During a biopsy, the doctor removes a very small amount of the lump. Then the lump is sent to a laboratory where it is examined for cancer cells.

(2) Mammograms are also used on large groups of women who have breasts which feel normal. These are called "screening mammograms". These mammograms are used to pick up tiny lumps which can't be felt.

Although screening mammograms can be useful, some people think they may not be safe for everyone. This is because even low dose X-rays may cause cancer to grow, if it is already there.

There is no proof that screening mammograms can save lives for women under fifty. They may be more useful for older women. Before you decide to have a mammogram, ask a lot of questions. Find out if there is a good reason for you to have one.

Examining your breasts is easy to do. Get into the habit of doing it every month. If you want help, ask your doctor or your public health nurse. After you know how to do it, show other women how. Show your daughters, your mother, your sisters and your friends how to examine their breasts too.

Breast self-examination is very important. It won't prevent you from getting cancer. But, it may stop you from dying from it.

Menopause

13

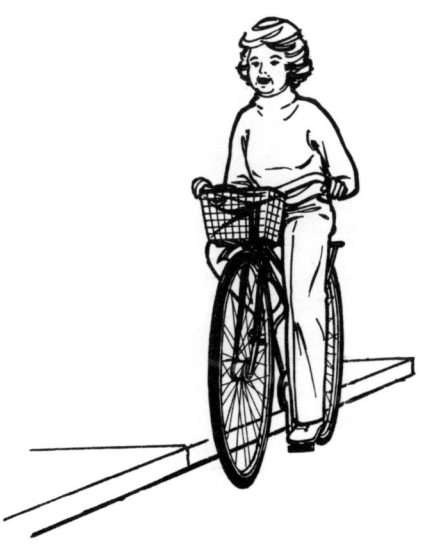

MENOPAUSE "THE CHANGE OF LIFE"

Menopause is a natural part of life which all women go through.

Some people have the wrong idea about menopause. Some people think that menopause makes women go a little crazy. Some people think that all women get depressed and fat during menopause. Others think that we lose all interest in sex after menopause. These ideas are wrong.

Menopause is not a medical problem or a disease. Most women go through menopause without too much trouble. Menopause will be much easier for you if you know what to expect, and if you know how to take care of yourself.

"What is menopause?"

Menopause is the time when our periods become irregular, until they finally stop altogether.

For nearly all women, menopause starts between age 40 and 55. For most women it ends when they are between 50 and 55. If you smoke, you may have an earlier menopause. If you have had a tubal ligation or a hysterectomy, you may have an earlier menopause.

Before menopause, your ovaries produce a regular amount of the hormone called estrogen. Estrogen causes the lining of your uterus (or womb) to grow every month. If you do not get pregnant, this lining is not needed. So, your body gets rid of it. It comes out of your body though your vagina. This is called "having your period".

During menopause, your ovaries start to produce less estrogen. When you start producing less estrogen, the lining of your uterus won't grow as thick. Then your periods will become lighter and irregular. Finally they will stop altogether.

Changes in your periods may be the first sign that your menopause is starting. Some women notice that their periods are lighter and shorter. Others find that theirs are longer and heavier. Some women skip a period now and again, and their periods become further apart. Others have their periods more often. Others go on having regular periods until they suddenly stop forever. All of these are normal.

Unusual Bleeding.

Some kinds of bleeding during menopause are not normal. Unusual bleeding can mean that something is wrong. Talk with your doctor if you have any bleeding like this:

1. Bleeding after having intercourse.
2. Very heavy bleeding or hemorrhaging with your period.
3. Large amounts of bleeding which are separate from your periods. If your periods are not regular, then it's hard to know when this is happening. Tell your doctor if this bleeding happens more than once in 3 weeks.
4. Very frequent periods. These may not be serious but they should be checked out.
5. Bleeding after six months or more have gone by since your last period.

Birth Control.

You can still get pregnant during your menopause. Some eggs are still released from your ovaries now and again. If you don't want to get pregnant, then you must still use birth control. You must also continue to use birth control for at least one whole year after your last period. The Pill is not a good method at this time. If you want more information on birth control, please read Chapter 9, <u>Birth Control</u>.

"How will my body change during menopause?"
Around the time of your menopause, your body will start to change. Some of these changes are due to having less estrogen. Other changes are due to aging.

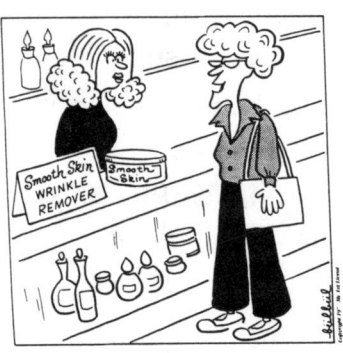

"What do you mean remove my wrinkles? I've earned every single one of them!"

© Bulbul, 1974

Common Changes During Menopause.

The most common changes during menopause are:
(1) Hot flashes
(2) Changes in your vagina
(3) Weakening of your bones

Each of these changes is described on the next pages, along with some suggestions for how to handle it.

Common Change #1: Hot Flashes.

"What are hot flashes?"

- Hot flashes are short, sudden heat waves that flow through your body. They can make you feel very over-heated, and they may make you sweat. Your face may turn red, or it may just feel like it is red. After a hot flash, you may feel chilled.

- Hot flashes can happen anytime, night or day. They can happen once a month or many times a day. When they happen at night, they can upset your sleep. If they often upset your sleep, then you may feel tired and miserable.

- Hot flashes are very common. They can be unpleasant, but they are not at all dangerous.

- Some women only have hot flashes for a few months. Others have them for a few years.

"What can I do about hot flashes?"

- First of all, don't be embarrassed by hot flashes. They are normal. Don't stay at home because of them. If you stay away from your friends, you may become lonely and depressed.

- Don't panic. They are normal and they will pass.

- Wear layers of clothes so that you can easily take off some clothes when a hot flash starts. At night, wear bed clothes that can easily be removed. Cotton clothes absorb sweat better than synthetics such as nylon or polyester.

- Carry something to use as a fan.
- Take deep breaths, in and out, slowly and regularly, when a hot flash starts.
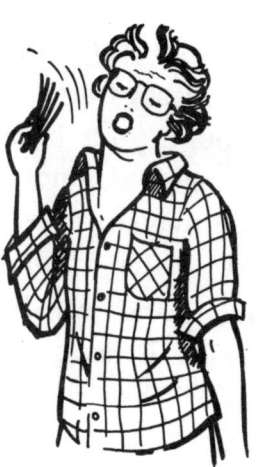
- Keep ice water nearby, and take a cold drink when you feel a hot flash starting.
- Keep the heat turned down in the winter.
- Don't take tranquillizers for hot flashes. They don't help, and they are addictive drugs.
- Try avoiding spicy foods and see if you have fewer hot flashes. This works for some women.
- Avoid tea, coffee and alcohol.
- Regular exercise helps some women to have fewer hot flashes.
- Join a Menopause Support Group. In this kind of group, you can get together with other women who are going through menopause. You can find out how other women handle their hot flashes and other problems. You can talk with other women, and give each other help and support. For many women, their support group is the best help of all.

These are all safe and easy ways to deal with hot flashes. They work for most women. However, if you have severe hot flashes which prevent you from working or sleeping, you might want to think about taking medication for a while.

There are two different drugs you could take for hot flashes: clonidine or estrogen.

Clonidine is a drug for high blood pressure. It can also help get rid of hot flashes, although it doesn't work for everyone. Clonidine only works well if you start taking it before your hot flashes are too severe.

Estrogen also helps hot flashes. However, when you stop taking it, your hot flashes may return. Also, estrogen is not safe for all women. Before you decide to take estrogen, you need to know if it is safe for you. Please read p. 392 in this chapter for more information about estrogen.

Common Change #2: Changes in Your Vagina.

"What changes will happen in my vagina?"

• Your vagina may be drier. During sex, your vagina may take longer to become wet, or it may not become very wet at all. The normal wetness in your vagina is called lubrication. If you have intercourse when your vagina is not lubricated, it can hurt. Your vagina can become irritated and then it may become infected.

• Your vagina may become tighter and less stretchable.

• Your vagina may become itchy.

• The lining of your vagina may become thinner. When it is thin, it may get tiny rips in it during intercourse.

Changes in your vagina do not mean the end of your sex life. Many women are as interested in sex after menopause as before. Some become much more interested. Others become less interested.

"What can I do about changes in my vagina?"

• Only have intercourse if your vagina is lubricated. If your vagina is not wet enough, you can buy a lubricating jelly in a drug store. Do not use petroleum jelly. It is not germ- free, and it does not wash away like water-soluble jelly does. Also, it weakens the latex in condoms and diaphragms.

- Some women find that having sex regularly makes them have more lubrication. Some women also find that masturbation helps this problem.

- If a lubricant doesn't help your dry vagina, estrogen creams can be very helpful. You do not use estrogen creams as a lubricant before sex. You need to apply estrogen to your vagina every day. Many women find that their vaginas are more comfortable after using the cream for a couple of weeks. After this, they only need to use the cream a few times a week. You need a prescription to buy estrogen cream.

There are some dangers in using estrogen. However, it is likely safer to use estrogen cream than to take estrogen pills. This is because less estrogen is absorbed into your body this way. If you want more information about estrogen, please read p. 392 in this chapter.

Common Change #3:
Osteoporosis, Weakening of Your Bones.

"What is osteoporosis?"

When we are young, our bones rebuild themselves all the time. As we get older, this rebuilding slows down. Some people's bones become quite thin and breakable. This is called "osteoporosis", which means bones with pores or holes in them.

Osteoporosis is a silent problem. You won't know that you have it at first. Then you might start to have pain in your lower back, or you might break your wrist after a small fall. 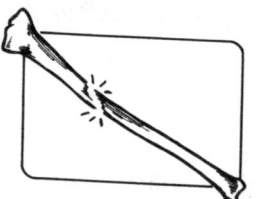 These are signs that your bones are not as strong as they should be. Osteoporosis can show up as early as middle-age.

Every woman will not get osteoporosis. Only about one in every four women will get osteoporosis.

After menopause, all woman have a greater risk of getting osteoporosis. Some women have even more risk than others.

These women are more likely to get osteoporosis:
- women who don't exercise.
- women who smoke.
- women who are thin and have small bones.
- women who don't get enough calcium in their food.

These women are also more likely to get osteoporosis:
- women who drink a lot of alcohol.
- women who drink a lot of tea, coffee and cola drinks.
- women who eat a great deal of meat.

"What can I do about osteoporosis?"
It is not easy to make weak bones strong again. So, the best way to deal with osteoporosis is to prevent it from ever happening. The best ways to prevent it are to exercise and to eat food containing lots of calcium.

Ways to prevent osteoporosis:
- **Exercise is a great way to prevent osteoporosis.** Exercise not only makes your muscles stronger. It also makes your bones stronger and thicker. You might enjoy a regular fitness class. Or, you might prefer riding your bike, or bowling, or swimming. These are all good exercises, and so is a simple 15-minute walk once a day.

If you already have osteoporosis, talk with your doctor before you start doing a lot of exercise. Some exercises can be harmful if you already have weak bones.

If you want more information on exercise, please read Chapter 4, <u>Being Active</u>.

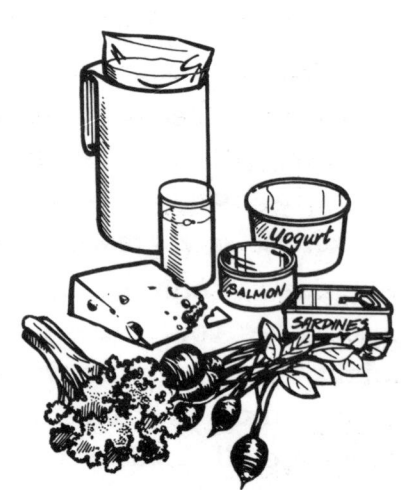

- **Eat lots of foods which contain calcium.**

Your body needs calcium to build strong bones. Most middle-aged and older women in Canada don't get nearly enough calcium every day. You can get a good supply of calcium by eating these foods:
- milk products (milk, cheese, yogurt)
- salmon and sardines (plus the bones)
- nuts (almonds, sunflower seeds)
- beans (kidney beans, chick peas)
- broccoli and other dark, leafy vegetables.
- tofu (bean curd)

Food is the best source of calcium. However, if you want to take calcium pills, choose pills which contain both calcium and magnesium. Your body needs a balance of these chemicals. Avoid dolomite. It often contains lead, which is dangerous. Check with your doctor before you take any new pills or medication.

• **Cut down on cigarettes, alcohol, coffee, tea, and cola drinks.**

• **You could take estrogen, but think about if first.** Estrogen may help to keep your bones stronger for a while. However, there are dangers to taking estrogen. You have to weigh both sides and make the choice that's best for you.

- On the one hand, estrogen makes your bones stay stronger for a longer time. However, when you stop taking it, your bones will start to lose calcium, sometimes very quickly.

- On the other hand, estrogen can be dangerous, especially if you still have your uterus. Because of its dangers, no one should take estrogen for the rest of her life.

Remember: only one out of every four women will develop osteoporosis. And, there are safe ways to prevent it. Think carefully about whether estrogen is a good choice for you. If you want to read more about taking estrogen, see p. 392 in this chapter.

Less Common Changes During Menopause.

Women sometimes notice other changes during menopause. The less common changes during menopause are:

(1) Depression
(2) Gaining Weight
(3) Constipation
(4) Stiffness
(5) Tiredness
(6) Incontinence, which means leaking some urine when you cough or sneeze.

No one has all of these problems.

Less Common Change #1: Depression.

Many women go through menopause without much trouble. However, some women become quite depressed during their menopause. Other women notice that their moods go up and down a lot.

If you are depressed, it may be hard to know if it is because of menopause, or because of other problems in your life.

Middle-age can be a difficult time. Menopause is often a time of lots of changes in your body and in your life. Besides your menopause, your children may be leaving home. You may also have the job of taking care of older parents. You may have your own health problems. You may not be getting enough sleep due to your hot flashes. You may be worrying that you are becoming less attractive. Any of these problems might make you feel depressed.

How we feel is often connected to the world we live in. We live in a world which doesn't show much respect or concern for middle-aged women and their problems. In many parts of the world, middle-aged women are respected and looked-up-to. But in Canada and the U.S., middle-aged women are not respected for their knowledge or for their experience.

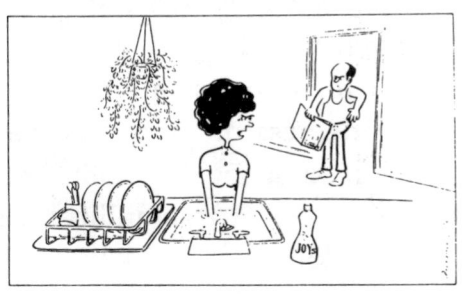

"No it's not menopausal depression. It's no pay, no sick leave, no pension, no identity."

© Bulbul, 1974

When a woman who is going through menopause is depressed, many people blame it on menopause. However, her depression may be partly because she is going through a hard time without enough help and support.

If you are feeling low, try not to stay home and worry. Try to get out of the house and keep busy. Remember to take care of yourself with good food, and a good balance of exercise and rest.

It can be a big help to talk with other women. You might be able to join a menopause support group where you can talk with other women. Some YWCAs run these support groups. A Women's Health Centre could also give you support and information.

A warning: Many doctors prescribe tranquillizers and sedatives to depressed, middle-aged women. These drugs are not useful for depression. In fact, they can make you more depressed. You may be taking a tranquillizer without knowing it. Some estrogen (hormone) pills also contain a tranquillizer which you may not want to be taking.

If you are depressed for a long time, you need some help. For more information about depression, please read Chapter 3, Depression.

Less Common Change #2: Gaining Weight.

As we get older, our bodies use food more slowly. Also, we need less food because we are usually less active. If we continue to eat as much food, we start to gain weight.

Most people in North America want to be thin. They think that thin is best, and thinner is even better. As a result, many women worry a lot about getting fat. Some women nearly starve themselves to stay thin. This is a big mistake.

All fat is not bad. However, more than 30 or 40 pounds of extra weight can cause health problems. The extra weight puts a strain on your heart. It can also make you more likely to get diabetes and high blood pressure.

If you have more then forty (40) extra pounds of fat, you should likely think about losing some weight. Less than forty extra pounds is less of a health risk. If your blood pressure is good, if you eat good food, 30 or even 40 pounds is not a big risk to your health.

Even if you don't like your extra fat, there may be a reason for it. During menopause, your body can use this fat to make some estrogen. This is useful when your overies are not making as much estrogen any more.

If you are worried about controlling your weight, the easiest way is to be more active. Exercise is all that many women have to do to control their weight. Exercise also helps them control their appetite. Exercise can prevent stiffness and aches and pains. It is also a great help for people who have trouble sleeping due to bad nerves. It also helps you get out of the house, and helps you feel good.

Eating good food - and cutting out junk food - also make a big difference to how well you feel.

If you want more information, please read Chapter 4, Being Active, and Chapter 5, Controlling Your Weight.

Less Common Change #3: Constipation.

Some women have problems with constipation as they get older. If you are often constipated, get more exercise, and change what you eat.

- Drink more water.
- Have some fruit or fruit juice, and vegetables every day.
- Eat more cereals, such as bran flakes.
- Eat whole grain breads.

Laxatives can be useful once in a while but they should not be used regularly. Changing what you eat is a safer and healthier thing to do.

Less Common Change #4: Stiffness, Aches and Pains.

Some women have stiffness and sore, aching joints during their menopause. The best cure for these pains is often careful exercise. Start off slowly. Ask your doctor or public health nurse for advice.

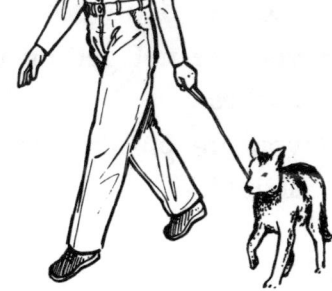

Walking is one of the best exercises. You don't need special equipment or training, and it's <u>very</u> cheap. Try walking downtown and taking the bus home. Try a short walk after supper. Ask a friend to go with you. Exercise will help you feel better both in your body and in your outlook. It will help control your appetite, and it will help you sleep better.

Less Common Change #5: Tiredness.

Some women have much more energy after menopause. However, some women feel more tired.

If you are tired all the time, then something is wrong. You may need to make some changes in your life, and take better care of yourself. If you can't figure out why you are so tired, talk with your doctor about it.

There are many common reasons that people feel tired. You may feel tired because:
- you are sick.
- you are depressed.
- you are not getting enough sleep because of hot flashes.
- you are pushing yourself to do more than you should.

You may be tired because:

- you are not getting enough exercise.
- you are not eating good regular meals.
- you are taking a drug that is making you feel tired. Both tranquillizers and alcohol can make you feel tired and depressed.
- you are drinking too much coffee or tea, or too many cola drinks which contain caffeine. These drinks wake you up at first, but they make you tired and edgy if you drink too much of them. They also prevent you from sleeping well.

Try to figure out what could be causing your tiredness. If you can't figure it out, get some help. Being tired all the time can make anyone miserable. Nearly always something can be done about it.

Less Common Change #6: Incontinence.

Incontinence means leaking some urine (pee) when you cough or sneeze.

Losing weight can help this problem. Exercises called "Kegel exercises" can also help. Exercises make muscles stronger, and Kegel exercises make the muscles stronger around the opening to your bladder and to your vagina.

How to do Kegel exercises:

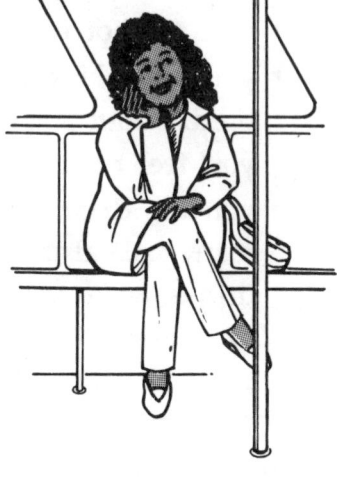

- Squeeze the muscles of your vagina as if you were trying to stop peeing. Continue squeezing and count to 5. Then relax and count to 5. Repeat this several times.

- The best time to practise these is when you are on the toilet. However, you can also do Kegel exercises anytime. You can do them while you are washing the dishes, or watching TV, or riding on the bus.

Other Changes.

Some women notice other changes during their menopause. Some of these are voice changes, sore breasts, headaches and a rapid heartbeat. You should talk with your doctor about these changes. They may be due to menopause, or they may be due to something else.

Medical Treatment For Menopause.

Menopause is a normal part of life. Most women can handle it by themselves without help from a doctor. However, some women have such serious symptoms that they go to their doctors for help and advice.

If you go to your doctor for help with your menopause, think about what kind of help you would like.

- You may just want to hear that your menopause symptoms are normal. If you know that they are normal, you may feel much better.
- You may want some advice about how to cope with menopause. Some doctors will suggest that you try some of the things you have read about in this book.
- You may want a medical way of handling your menopause. You may want to know more about taking hormones, or about having a hysterectomy. Most women do not need a medical treatment for their menopause.

Taking Hormones.

During menopause our bodies start to make less of the hormone called estrogen. Many doctors think women should replace this estrogen by taking estrogen shots or pills.

Your doctor will give you estrogen by itself, or with another hormone called progesterone. Estrogen is usually prescribed as pills or shots. It is also prescribed in a patch which is applied to your skin. It can also be prescribed as a cream for your vagina.

Millions of women take estrogen because it has some benefits for some women. However, taking estrogen can be risky for some women. If you are thinking about taking hormones, compare the risks with the benefits.

Benefits of taking estrogen:

- Estrogen is helpful if you have your ovaries removed in a complete hysterectomy. After your operation, you will not be able to produce much estrogen. Doctors call this a "surgical menopause". Taking estrogen can be useful until you reach the age of normal menopause — about age 50.

If you have a high risk of having osteoporosis, you may need to keep taking estrogen after you turn 50. (Please read p. 378.) A bone-density test will help you decide what to do.

- Estrogen is useful for keeping calcium in your bones. Calcium is necessary for strong bones. However, when you stop taking estrogen, your bones will start to lose calcium. Sometimes this happens very quickly.

- Estrogen cream is useful if your vagina is very dry. It can make your vagina wetter, and this makes sex much moı comfortable.

Estrogen cream is likely safer to use than estrogen pills because you likely won't need it for very long. (If you want more information about estrogen creams, please read p. 377 in this chapter.

- Estrogen is useful for hot flashes. However, when you stop taking estrogen, your hot flashes may return. This is one reason why many women decide to cope with hot flashes without estrogen.

> No matter what anyone tells you, estrogen will not keep you young forever.

Risks of taking estrogen:

- All women have some risk of getting cancer in their uterus (or womb). However, if you take estrogen by itself for more than two years, you are 4 times more likely to get this cancer. The longer you take it, the greater the risk.
  Because this cancer risk is so high, doctors often prescribe progesterone with the estrogen. If you take both progesterone and estrogen, your risk of getting cancer is much less. In fact, you end up with less risk of cancer in your uterus than a woman who is not taking any estrogen. However, there are other reasons for not taking estrogen.

- Estrogen can increase your risk of having breast cancer.

- Estrogen can make fibroids in your uterus develop and grow more quickly. (Fibroids are growths which are not cancer. They can cause heavy bleeding.)

- Estrogen is dangerous for women who have the following health problems:

1. You must not take estrogen if you have had:
   - a stroke or high blood pressure
   - cancer of the breast or uterus
   - liver disease
   - blood-clotting problems
   - unusual vaginal bleeding
   - breast cysts
2. You must not take estrogen if your mother or sister had breast cancer.
3. You must not take estrogen if you or your mother took D.E.S.

   D.E.S. stands for Di-ethyl-stilbestrol. D.E.S. is a drug which contains estrogen. It was used between 1941 and 1971. Doctors gave it to pregnant women because it was supposed to prevent miscarriages.

   Now we know that D.E.S. was harmful to some of the babies of these women. These problems don't show up until the people are teenagers or adults.

Women whose mothers took D.E.S. are called "D.E.S. daughters". D.E.S. daughters may have trouble getting pregnant. They may have more miscarriages, and more problems with their menstrual periods. A small number of D.E.S. daughters get cancer of the vagina and the cervix.

If you were born between 1941 and 1971, try to find out if your mother took D.E.S.. Ask her if she took any pills or had any shots to prevent a miscarriage. (It may be hard to find out what drugs she took. She may not remember, and her medical records may have been destroyed.)

If you think you are a D.E.S. daughter, you should not take more estrogen. You also need to be examined by a doctor who has experience with D.E.S.. The doctor will look for any problems which may have been caused by D.E.S..

4. You should talk with your doctor before taking estrogen if you have any of these health problems:

- diabetes
- varicose veins
- migraine headaches
- phlebitis
- gall bladder attacks
- fibroids in your uterus

You can see estrogen is not for everyone. Before you take it, compare the risks with the benefits. Make sure you have a good reason to take it. Make sure there are no serious reasons why you should not take it. If you decide to take estrogen, here are some rules for how to use it more safely.

Rules for using estrogen more safely.

1. Take the smallest amount of estrogen for the shortest time. Think of estrogen as a temporary way to help you.

2. While you are taking estrogen, have a check-up after 6 months, and have a Pap test every year.

3. When you go for your regular checkups, ask your doctor about the latest research on hormones.

4. Be sure to examine your breasts carefully every month.

5. Pay attention to any changes in your body, and tell your doctor about them. Some of them may be danger signs.

Call your doctor at once if you have any of these danger signs:
- Bleeding or spotting from your vagina other than your period. (If you are taking both estrogen and progesterone, you will continue to have periods, even if you are going through menopause. This makes it very hard to know if you are having unusual bleeding. Ask your doctor about this.)
- Chest pain or difficulty in breathing
- Severe headaches
- Changes in how well you can see
- Pains in the lower part of your leg
- A breast lump
- Yellowing of your skin or eyes

DANGER SIGNS

Remember, women have coped for many years without estrogen. We didn't need to take hormones when our periods were starting. So, most of us don't need hormones when our periods are ending either. There are other, safer ways to deal with most of the problems of menopause. Before you choose estrogen, try the safer ways first.

Hysterectomy.

A hysterectomy is an operation which removes your uterus (or womb). Often only your uterus is removed. Sometimes your tubes and ovaries are also taken out.

Many women have a hysterectomy during their menopause. Sometimes the operation is necessary, and sometimes it is not. Some people think that one third of all hysterectomies are unnecessary.

If you have one of these problems, then you likely need a hysterectomy:
- cancer of the uterus, ovaries or vagina
- severe bleeding that cannot be controlled by drugs or by D. and C.'s (Read p. 401 for more information.)
- a severe, uncontrollable infection in the uterus, called Pelvic Inflammatory Disease, or P.I.D..
  A hysterectomy should only be done as a last resort for P.I.D. because the operation can make the infection worse. (If you want more information on P.I.D., please read p. 263, in Chapter 8, Sex.)

If you have one of these problems, then you likely do not need a hysterectomy:
- menopause
- simple menstrual pain.

If you want an abortion or if you want to be sterilized, you do <u>not</u> need a hysterectomy. (Tubal ligations and vasectomies are safer and easier ways to be sterilized.)

Hysterectomy is a serious operation. After a hysterectomy, some women are depressed and very tired for a long time. Others have much less interest in sex, and they cannot easily have orgasms any more. Some women can take as long as two years to recover from a hysterectomy. A women's support-group can be a big help at this time.

Think carefully before you decide to have a hysterectomy. Unless your life is in danger, or unless you have terrible pain that can't be treated, get a second opinion from another doctor.

- Ask your doctor whether or not your ovaries are going to be removed in the operation. If your ovaries are healthy, they do not have to be removed.
- Ask your doctors what else you could do for your problem, such as an operation to remove only the fibroids, not your whole uterus.
- Ask them if you should have a "D. and C." first.

The D. and C.

A D. and C. is a much simpler operation than a hysterectomy. During a D. and C., the doctor scrapes away the lining of your uterus with a long, spoon-like instrument. This instrument is put into your uterus through your vagina. No cuts are made. Sometimes this is all that you need to control heavy bleeding.

Hysterectomy and Menopause.

Some women think that they won't go through menopause if they have had a hysterectomy. This is not true. All women go through menopause whenever their ovaries start producing less estrogen. If you had a hysterectomy, then the time of your menopause depends on whether or not your ovaries were removed in the operation.

(1) If you only had your uterus taken out, and not your ovaries, then your ovaries will likely continue to produce estrogen. They will stay active until you are between 40 and 50. Then your ovaries will start to produce less estrogen. This will be the beginning of your menopause.

Without a uterus, you will have a harder time knowing when your menopause is starting. Many women know that menopause is starting when their periods become irregular. However, you won't have periods anymore, so you won't have this common first sign of menopause. However, you may notice hot flashes or some other sign that menopause is beginning.

(2) If both your uterus and your ovaries were taken out, then your menopause began right after your operation. This is a "surgical menopause". You might have this operation at any age, but it is more often done if you are in your 40's or 50's.

When your ovaries are removed, your estrogen level drops quite suddenly. This sudden drop in estrogen can be quite hard to handle. It takes time to get used to.

Many women take estrogen to help their bodies adjust. The estrogen in the pills or shots or patches replaces some of your body's estrogen. It replaces the estrogen which their ovaries can't produce any more.

Estrogen may be useful for a while, but you will not need to take for the rest of your life. Eventually you should be able to stop taking it altogether.

Whatever your doctor suggests, remember that you have the right to ask questions and to get answers that you can understand. If your doctor suggests that you have a hysterectomy, you have the right to a second opinion from a different doctor. The more you know, the easier it is to decide what is best.

Many people still think of menopause as the end of a woman's usefulness. This is not true. Menopause is the end of only one thing - menstrual periods. During and after your menopause you can still continue to work, think, and enjoy life. If you no longer have children to care for, you may now have time for what you want to do. You may have time to learn new things, or time to try something you never had time for before, or time just to relax.

After menopause, you may still have one third of your life left ahead of you. For many women it is a new beginning. Middle-age can be - and should be - a very good part of your life.